Neuro Spinal Surgery
Operative Techniques
Micro Lumbar Discectomy
The Gold Standard

Neuro Spinal Surgery Operative Techniques
Micro Lumbar Discectomy
The Gold Standard

JKBC Parthiban
MCh (Neurosurgery) FNS (Japan)
Senior Consultant (Neurosurgery and Spine Neurosurgery)
Kovai Medical Center and Hospital
Coimbatore, Tamil Nadu, India

Forewords
John Ebnezar
S Balaji Pai

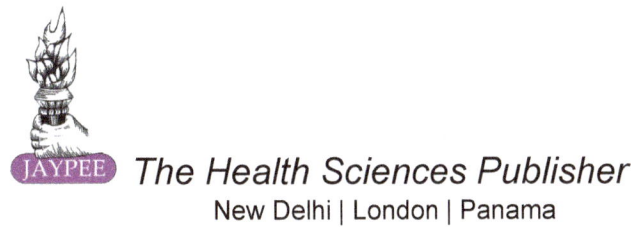

JAYPEE The Health Sciences Publisher
New Delhi | London | Panama

Jaypee Brothers Medical Publishers (P) Ltd.

Headquarters
Jaypee Brothers Medical Publishers (P) Ltd.
4838/24, Ansari Road, Daryaganj
New Delhi 110 002, India
Phone: +91-11-43574357
Fax: +91-11-43574314
E-mail: jaypee@jaypeebrothers.com

Overseas Offices

J.P. Medical Ltd.
83, Victoria Street, London, SW1H 0HW (UK)
Phone: +44-20 3170 8910
Fax: +44(0) 20 3008 6180
e-mail: info@jpmedpub.com

Jaypee-Highlights Medical Publishers Inc.
City of Knowledge, Building 235, 2nd Floor
Clayton, Panama City, Panama
Phone: +1 507-301-0496
Fax: +1 507-301-0499
E-mail: cservice@jphmedical.com

Jaypee Brothers Medical Publishers (P) Ltd.
17/1-B, Babar Road, Block-B
Shaymali, Mohammadpur
Dhaka-1207, Bangladesh
Mobile: +08801912003485
E-mail: jaypeedhaka@gmail.com

Jaypee Brothers Medical Publishers (P) Ltd.
Bhotahity, Kathmandu, Nepal
Phone: +977-9741283608
E-mail: kathmandu@jaypeebrothers.com

Website: www.jaypeebrothers.com
Website: www.jaypeedigital.com

© 2017, Jaypee Brothers Medical Publishers

The views and opinions expressed in this book are solely those of the original contributor(s)/author(s) and do not necessarily represent those of editor(s) of the book.

All rights reserved. No part of this publication may be reproduced, stored or transmitted in any form or by any means, electronic, mechanical, photocopying, recording or otherwise, without the prior permission in writing of the publishers.

All brand names and product names used in this book are trade names, service marks, trademarks or registered trademarks of their respective owners. The publisher is not associated with any product or vendor mentioned in this book.

Medical knowledge and practice change constantly. This book is designed to provide accurate, authoritative information about the subject matter in question. However, readers are advised to check the most current information available on procedures included and check information from the manufacturer of each product to be administered, to verify the recommended dose, formula, method and duration of administration, adverse effects and contraindications. It is the responsibility of the practitioner to take all appropriate safety precautions. Neither the publisher nor the author(s)/editor(s) assume any liability for any injury and/or damage to persons or property arising from or related to use of material in this book.

This book is sold on the understanding that the publisher is not engaged in providing professional medical services. If such advice or services are required, the services of a competent medical professional should be sought.

Every effort has been made where necessary to contact holders of copyright to obtain permission to reproduce copyright material. If any have been inadvertently overlooked, the publisher will be pleased to make the necessary arrangements at the first opportunity.

Inquiries for bulk sales may be solicited at: jaypee@jaypeebrothers.com

Neuro Spinal Surgery Operative Techniques—Micro Lumbar Discectomy: The Gold Standard

First Edition: **2017**

ISBN: 978-93-5270-050-9

Printed at

Dedicated to
Professor PS Ramani

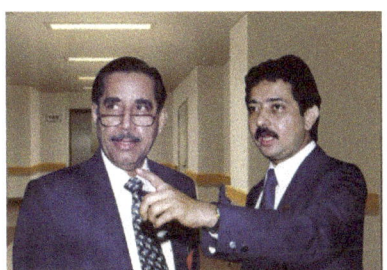

My tete-a-tete with Professor PS Ramani
during the Neurotrauma Conference in Cochin, 1995

Foreword

Low backache is a global malady. Disc problems are a big contributor to this common problem. Surgery becomes a necessity when conservative methods fail. Open lumbar discectomy (OLD) was the preferred technique till micro lumbar discectomy (MLD) came into vogue. With its advantages, it soon became the gold standard which is true even to this day. Though newer techniques in the form of endoscopic lumbar discectomy (ELD), percutaneous lumbar discectomy 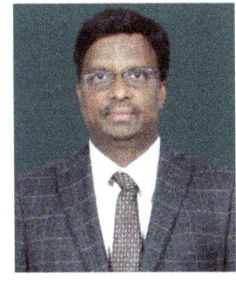 (PLD) and other innovative techniques were later introduced, MLD has managed to remain on the top. But MLD is not every surgeon's cup of tea like the OLD. It has a steep learning curve and requires special surgical instrumentation and skills. Not everyone gets an opportunity to update and learn this skill by visiting centers of surgical excellence under masters. Though there are many books on this subject, not many teach the basics and complexities of this demanding technique. This is where Dr Parthiban's book effectively fills up these lacunae.

This book has 10 chapters and is very well written. The language is very easy to understand, simple and lucid. The first chapter on anatomy is made attractive and interesting by good diagrams, the second chapter deals with the much neglected preoperative preparations on which the success of the surgery is based. The third chapter is the soul of the book—it is of great use to the young spine surgeons as it deals with various case scenarios with the best possible operative techniques to handle each and every challenging situation that one encounters in a day-to-day practice. The subsequent chapters deal with on-table complications and ways to avoid and get out of them; steps to prevent epidural fibrosis, which can become a troublesome problem to handle, epidural medications to counter it. Chapters on instrumentation, microscopes and magnifying loupes stress the role of instruments in the successful surgical outcomes. He summarizes the whole technique very well in the final chapter. Needless to say, Dr Parthiban has done a very decent job on this technique, and everyone who reads this book will no longer find MLD a difficult summit to scale.

He has put years of hard work and knowledge into making this book. He is a personal friend of mine and is an eminent neurosurgeon of international repute. He is a big name in his field and has several innovations and newer implants on his name. He is extremely hardworking and dedicated to his profession and skill. What makes him stand apart from others is his humility, grace, willingness to learn and a burning desire to propagate and spread knowledge. He has overcome many personal and professional challenges to reach where he has reached today. Above all, he is an excellent human being; unassuming and uncomplicated, which is a rarity in today's dog-eat-dog world.

I congratulate him for this stupendous effort and wish to see many more books from his pen. I, being an author and writer myself, know how difficult it is to write a single chapter, let alone a book. It is very aptly said 'the pen is mightier than the sword', but it requires more might to tame the pen! In fact, his first foray into writing began with a chapter on spine surgery, which he contributed to my book *Step-by-step Operative Techniques,* a few years ago. That chapter was very much appreciated by the readers and now he has gone solo with this book and I am sure that this book will be a great success and become a landmark book on the art of MLD.

I wish him all the best and pray to the Almighty to give him health, wealth and happiness that he richly deserves. It is an absolute pleasure and honor to write a Foreword for his maiden book and I thank him for choosing me to do the honors.

Padma Shri John Ebnezar
PhD (Yoga) MD (Ortho-Hons) MBBS D Ortho DNB (Ortho) MNAMS (Ortho)
Sports Medicine (Australia), IOA-INOR Fellow (United Kingdom)
Consulting Orthopedic, Sports Specialist, Spine Surgeon and Wholistic Orthopedic Expert
Geriatric Orthopedic Surgeon
Founder President, Geriatric Orthopedic Society of India (GOSI)
Founder Director, Geriatric Orthopedic Association of India (GOAI)
Medical Superintendent, CV Raman General Hospital, Indiranagar
CEO, Parimala Health Care Services
Chief Orthopedic and Spine Surgeon, Dr John's Orthopedic Center
Bengaluru, Karnataka, India

Foreword

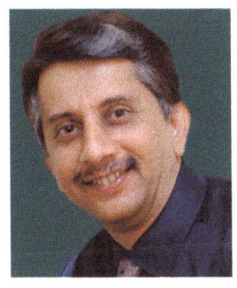

It is indeed a privilege and honor to write a Foreword for this book written by Dr Parthiban, who has been a teacher, friend, philosopher and guide to me since my resident years. Microscopic surgery is an essential aspect of neurosurgery and spinal surgery. Micro lumbar discectomy remains the gold standard against which the other minimally invasive disc surgeries are compared. Micro lumbar discectomy is the first step in the training of all neurosurgery and spinal surgery residents. It affords all residents training and confidence to proceed further in their neurosurgical career. Hence, the importance of this surgical procedure cannot be underestimated. I appreciate and admire the efforts of Dr Parthiban in bringing out this book after recognizing the importance of this surgical procedure in the careers of neuro and spine surgeons.

The book is spread out in an organized fashion. Starting with the applied anatomy, the author takes the reader through the importance of preoperative planning, especially positioning. The book then deals, in length and detail, with the operative techniques of micro lumbar discectomy. The quality and the importance devoted to figures and illustrations is truly commendable. The 'surgical tricks' incorporated by the author are truly helpful. Accompanying lateral canal stenosis is always a surgical challenge and the book details how to tackle this problem, including the disc migration issue. The problem of recurrent disc prolapse which is not discussed frequently in the literature and holds importance to the senior surgeons, is also handled adeptly in the book. Far lateral disc prolapse is uncommon and generally not encountered by the residents and even some consultants. This book serves as a surgical guide for surgeons who attempt this uncommon problem. The author also devotes a section in the book to intraoperative complications, wherein the author describes the common intraoperative complications and methods to manage them. Although the "man behind the machine" is important, it is also imperative that the surgeon is provided with the basic surgical instruments and paraphernalia required for this surgery. This is also effectively dealt with in the book. A chapter on the common postoperative complications could have been included and I am sure the future editions will incorporate it.

I find this book a treatise in the important surgical procedure of micro lumbar discectomy and recommend it to all the residents and junior consultants of neurosurgery and spinal surgery, which it has been targeted towards. I also congratulate Dr Parthiban for his stellar efforts.

S Balaji Pai
Head
Department of Neurosurgery
Bangalore Medical College and Research Institute
Bengaluru, Karnataka, India

Preface

Why micro lumbar discectomy (MLD) is still the most preferred technique for lumbar disc prolapse? Why other modes of treatment are not practiced widely? The answer is simple—MLD is an offshoot of the yesteryears' most popular technique laminectomy that was widely practiced by neurosurgeons for many years and hence is easy to learn and perform using microscope. Many neurosurgeons easily learn this technique by virtue of their basic training in microsurgery during resident period. Hence, any surgeon, who likes to do MLD, should get trained in handling of microscopes and microsurgery. Microscopes provide good light illumination, clarity and required magnification with no visual distortions. Head lamps and loupes may fall short of comfort to the surgeons. Also, assistant and scrub nurses can observe and help in the procedure with microscopes that are lacking in loupe assistance.

Micro lumbar discectomy has definitely surpassed the results provided by the vintage laminectomy. In the recent years, many other techniques are getting into practice by well-trained surgeons, viz. percutaneous endoscopic discectomies. In this technique, the learning curve is steep and the benefits are yet to be proved better than MLD, though a few specialists claim so. It may be true in a master's hand that his technique provides better result than MLD. It is like a fine violinist bringing out the best music from his instrument. But it is not easy to become a violinist in the first place itself. Hence, there need not be any argument in claiming whose music is better and which gives the best result in a given setup. A violinist and a *veena* (lute) master can provide the best music with their respective instruments and need not be compared. What we need is a good music, a good nerve root decompression and long-lasting pain-free period. Here, I have no intention of discussing anything else other than detailing the value of MLD in the management of lumbar discectomy.

I have been practicing this technique since 1991, and I found it versatile, and it can be applied in all types of lumbar disc prolapses, except in rare situations, where there are degenerative canal stenosis of severe degree. Once practiced systematically by choosing simple cases in the beginning, the surgeon can master it over a short period. As in all surgeries, one should understand the planes of dissection and respect the stability of facet joints. Once tasted the best results, surgeons practicing MLD may not shift to other techniques unless warranted or forced to do due to peer pressure to adopt a newer one to keep oneself in front line of practice.

I have written this book with the aim of providing an opportunity for those young neurosurgeons who had no guidance in their learning period, and for the surgeons, who wanted to shift from laminectomy to MLD.

Books are not written to be followed blindly. Surgeons are requested to go through it leisurely; but, at the same time, cautiously, and then practice with care and guidance. In case of doubt, no time should be wasted to communicate with me for clarification. My best wishes to all who are going to be benefitted by this small book.

Finally, we live here to transfer our knowledge to others for the benefit of mankind.

JKBC Parthiban

Acknowledgments

Nothing is possible without my patients, who had faith in me. This book is no exception. I am greatly indebted to all of them who extended their cooperation for this venture.

Many thanks go to my mentor, Professor PS Ramani, for teaching me the basic techniques in micro lumbar discectomy in 1991.

My thanks go to—

The staff and management of Medical Trust Hospital, Cochin; Global Hospital, Chennai; and Kovai Medical Center and Hospital, Coimbatore, for their support.

My nursing staff and theater technicians for their whole-hearted involvement.

Mr N Krishnamurthy and Mr S Sivakumar for helping in positioning, bolster maintenance and microscope recording and retrieving data.

Dr K Rajendran, neuroanesthetist, for personally setting up the bolsters for all my patients ever since it was introduced and in titration of epidural medication.

Mr Oliver and Mr Sam for designing the prototypes of double-hook retractors.

Dr Shanthanam for collecting my case studies and microscopic pictures and data for this subject.

Dr John Ebnezar for having given permission to use some of the clinical materials from the Section 3: Spine, Chapter 15: Lumbar Disc Surgery, contributed by me in the book *Operative Orthopaedics*.

M/s Jaypee Brothers Medical Publishers (P) Ltd., New Delhi, India, especially to Shri Jitendar P Vij (Group Chairman), Mr Ankit Vij (Group President), Mrs Chetna Malhotra Vohra (Associate Director–Content Strategy) for her immense help in shaping and bringing out the book in this present shape, Mr Sabarish Menon (Commissioning Editor), who was in constant touch until the last moves were made to get the book completed, Mr KK Raman (Production Manager), Mr Sunil Kr Dogra (Production Coordinator) for giving the finishing touch to the book, Mr Ashutosh Srivastava (Asstt Editor), Mr Ashutosh Pathak (Proofreader), Mr Manoj Pahuja (Sr Graphic Designer), and Mr Vinod Sharma (Typesetter).

Contents

1. **Basic Applied Anatomy**   1
   - Lumbar Disc *1*
   - Interlaminar Space *2*
   - Ligamentum Flavum *3*
   - Epidural Space *3*
   - Epidural Veins *5*
   - Lumbar Neural Foramen *5*
   - Far-lateral Space *6*
   - Disc Prolapses and Sites *6*

2. **Preoperative Preparations**   10
   - Positioning *10*
   - Level Marking *13*
   - Preparation of Operating Site *15*

3. **Operative Techniques with Case Examples**   16
   - Interlaminar Approach *16*
     - Lateral Disc Prolapse—Lower Level *16*
     - Centrolateral Large Disc Prolapse with Lateral Canal Stenosis *52*
     - Lateral Disc Prolapse—Upper Level *75*
   - Migration *84*
     - Inferior Migration of Large Fragments—Central and Lateral *84*
     - Inferior Migration—Central *92*
     - Superior Migration—Lateral *98*
   - Recurrent Disc Prolapse *105*
     - Recurrent Disc Prolapse (Acute and Small) *105*
     - Recurrent Disc Prolapse (Chronic and Large) *113*
     - Far-lateral Disc Prolapse (Shoulder Approach) *123*
     - Far-lateral Disc Prolapse (Axillary Approach) *130*
     - Foraminotomy and Discectomy (Axillary Approach) *131*

4. **On-table Complications**   136
   - Dural Tear *136*
   - Epidural Venous Bleed *139*

5.	Steps to Prevent Epidural Fibrosis	142
6.	Epidural Medications	143
7.	Micro Lumbar Double-hook Retractors	144
8.	Instruments	148
9.	Microscopes and Magnifying Loupes	155
10.	Final Thoughts	157

Index *161*

Introduction

The principle of micro lumbar discectomy (MLD) is to achieve adequate decompression of the clinically correlating nerve root under compression due to prolapsed disc fragments, thickened ligamentum flavum, crowded facet joints, osteophytes, etc. through a small skin incision without jeopardizing the spinal segmental stability. Ideally speaking, micro lumbar discectomy (MLD) is microsurgical decompression of lumbar nerve root (MDLNR). Since MLD is a commonly used terminology, I continue to address it the same way in this book. The other names for this procedure with minimal changes are lumbar micro discectomy (LMD) and fenestration, etc.

I learned this technique from Dr Ramani in 1991, and subsequently mastered it and later changed a few techniques to my comfort. This book covers entire variety of techniques that are used for decompressing the lumbar nerve roots by removing disc prolapses at various sites through minimal access and by preserving the motion segment. The importance of bolsters, use of double-hook retractors and microscopes, managing epidural hemorrhage and dural tear, are covered in detail. Large numbers of high-definition microsurgical pictures of surgical procedures supported by illustrative line diagrams drawn by me, provide ample knowledge to young surgeons to follow up with ease and master this very effective surgical treatment of symptomatic lumbar disc prolapse.

CHAPTER 1

Basic Applied Anatomy

LUMBAR DISC

Lumbar disc, between two adjacent vertebral bodies, has two major components viz. Annulus and nucleus pulposus. Annulus is thick with its horizontal and vertical fibers and merges with cartilage of vertebral body **(Figs 1.1 and 1.2)**. It has sensory nerve fibers that supply annulus. Nucleus pulposus is made up of glycoproteins and is thick. It is avascular.

During degeneration, water content in nucleus is depleted and the nucleus changes its texture, bulges inside the compound of annulus which, in turn, bulges thus changing the natural contour of whole disc **(Fig. 1.3)**. The degenerated disc materials then extrude under pressure through the fissures in annulus layer by layer. When the fissures enlarge to become rents the degenerated disc material extrudes through them into the canal. The disc material may be in continuity or may stay below the posterior longitudinal ligament or may get detached from the intradiscal part and even migrate superiorly or inferiorly.

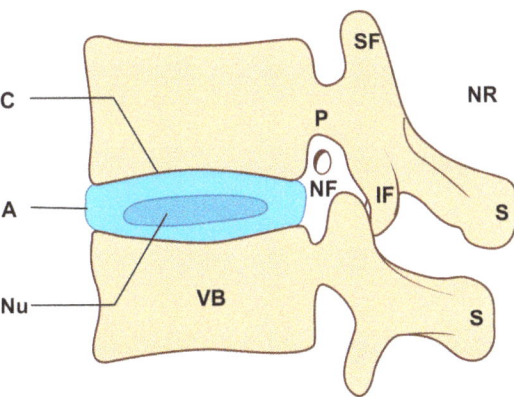

Fig. 1.1 Lumbar disc
Abbreviations: A, annulus; C, cartilage; IF, inferior facet; NF, neural foramen; NR, nerve root; Nu, nucleus pulposus; P, pedicle, S, spinous process; SF, superior facet; VB, vertebral body

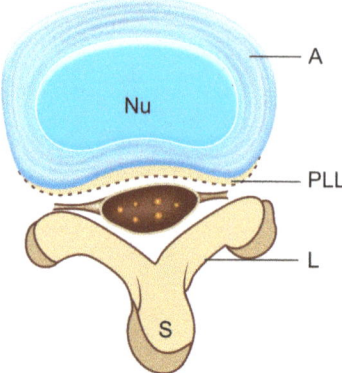

Fig. 1.2 Lumbar disc
Abbreviations: A, annulus; L, lamina; PLL, posterior longitudinal ligament; Nu, nucleus pulposus; S, spinous process

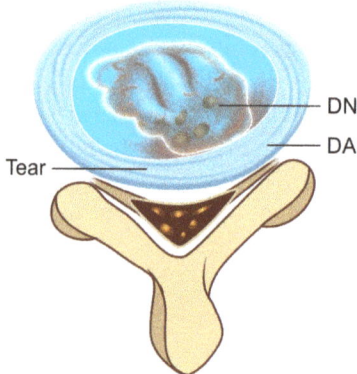

Fig. 1.3 Disc bulge
Abbreviations: DA, deformed annulus; DN, degenerated nucleus pulposus

Depending on the way the disc bulges and the disc materials extrude and are classified in many ways. However, in practice and during decision making for surgical intervention, one needs to know the following-anatomical location of extruded disc, shape of the disc bulge, volume of spinal canal, thickened ligaments, facet joints and laminae.

INTERLAMINAR SPACE

Assessment of interlaminar space is important before surgical planning. This space is widest at L_5/S_1 level and becomes narrow at higher levels **(Fig. 1.4)**. On flexion of lumbar spine, interlaminar space widens further facilitating a good surgical corridor. In severe degenerative spine with hypertrophic facet joints, this space is very narrow and does not widen on flexion.

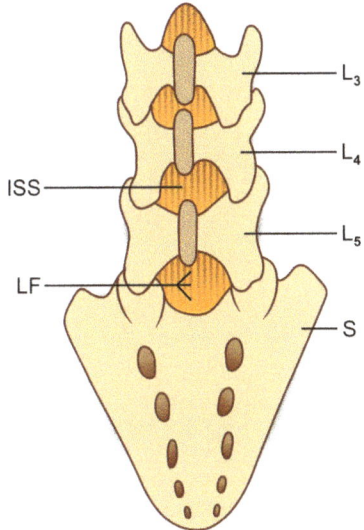

Fig. 1.4 Interlaminar space
Abbreviations: ISS, interspinous space; LF, ligamentum flavum; S, sacrum

LIGAMENTUM FLAVUM

Ligamentum flavum is a thick ligament that drapes the entire posterior border of the lumbar canal. It is light yellow in color and the fibers are craniocaudal in direction and are very much elastic. Inferiorly it is attached to the superior border of lamina of inferior vertebra; and superiorly, it is attached to the ventral (under) surface of superior lamina **(Fig. 1.5)**. Laterally, they drape the facet joints on their ventral surface thus forming the posterior border of the lateral canal.

Since the ligament is elastic, they are stretched well in flexion and are under tension. In extension of lumbar spine, they are lax and look thickened. In degenerated lumbar segment, when the intervertebral disc space is reduced leading to settlement, the ligamentum flavum gets buckled thus causing stenosis. The thickened ligament is actually the folded and buckled ligament in severely degenerated lumbar segment. Prolapsed and bulged annulus increases the agony. Hence meticulously removing the buckled ligament is very important in achieving dorsal decompression before completing discectomy.

EPIDURAL SPACE

Epidural space is filled with fat and when the canal is free, dorsal dura can be seen lax and pulsatile. Epidural veins (plexus) can be seen on the dorsum,

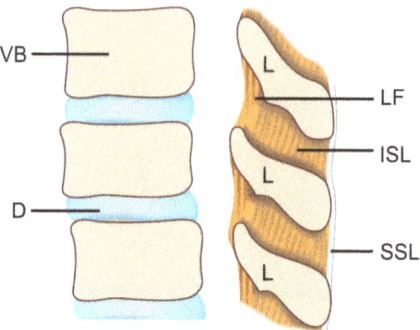

Fig. 1.5 Ligamentum flavum
Abbreviations: D, disc; LF, ligamentum flavum; ISL, interspinous ligament; SSL, supraspinous ligament; VB, vertebral body

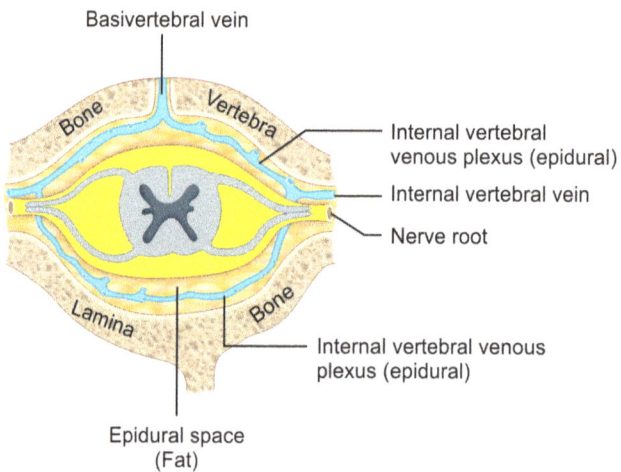

Fig. 1.6 Batson's venous plexus (Epidural)

ventral and lateral canal (**Fig. 1.6**). In acute disc prolapses and in small disc prolapses, the epidural space may look free. However, the nerve root sleeve may be seen stretched over the disc prolapse and, sometimes, it is hard to find the dural sleeve edge. In chronic disc prolapses and in long-term degenerative canal stenosis, the dura gets thinned out and has the tendency to get damaged easily. One can see the subarachnoid cerebrospinal fluid and the cauda equina fibers through the thinned out dura. Change in color of the dura determines the severity of compression. Normally, dura is white in color with small vessels running over the dura and nerve roots.

Basic Applied Anatomy | 5

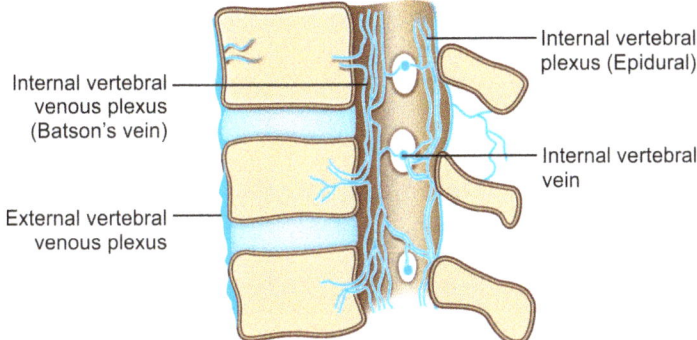

Fig. 1.7 Batson's venous plexus (Lumbar canal venous drainage)

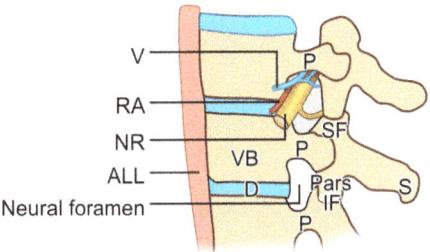

Fig. 1.8 Neural foramen
Abbreviations: ALL, anterior longitudinal ligament; D, disc; IF, inferior facet; NR, nerve root; P, pedicle; RA, radicular artery; S, spinous process; SF, superior facet; V, internal vertebral vein; VB, vertebral body

EPIDURAL VEINS

Epidural veins are dilated and engorged above the level of disc prolapse. Often they are encountered in the lateral canal and should be inspected well. The Batson's plexus is a large system that drains the lumbar canal venous drainage **(Fig. 1.7)**. Some lacunae are large and are seen anterior to ventral dura at lumbar region. Many times after removal of large disc, significant epidural bleed will be encountered. This needs patience to control them and the bleed signifies good decompression too.

LUMBAR NEURAL FORAMEN

Intervertebral space through which the spinal nerves pass out to form the lumbar plexus **(Fig. 1.8)**. Foramen is formed by the pedicles above and below, the posterior wall of the cephalad vertebral body and disc anteriorly and the pars interarticularis posteriorly. Lateral margin is formed by the lateral edge of pars and medial margin by an imaginary line connecting the medial border of adjacent pedicles. Foramen looks like an ear viewing from side.

FAR-LATERAL SPACE

This is the space that is lateral to the foramen and is bordered by the posterior longitudinal ligament covering the cephalad vertebra and disc anteriorly and the ligamentum flavum and intertransverse ligament posteriorly. The facet joint overhangs the caudal aspect of the lateral space, partially covering the disc posteriorly. This space contains the emerging nerve root, ganglion, radicular artery, radicular vein, epidural vein and plexus **(Fig. 1.9)**.

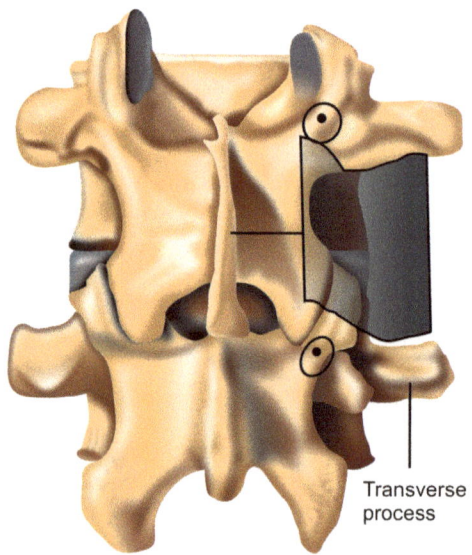

Fig. 1.9 Far lateral space—lateral to neural foramen

DISC PROLAPSES AND SITES

Approach to prolapsed lumbar disc depends on its site and its correlation with the symptoms. Though many classifications are in literature in practice, the surgeon has to plan the best approach to excise them and achieve satisfactory nerve root decompression. Degenerative disc bulge is common and the annulus bulges thus encroaching the spinal canal causing central canal stenosis, lateral canal stenosis, unilateral and, sometimes, bilateral. This, along with degenerative facet joints and buckling ligamentum flavum can cause various symptoms, viz; sciatica, cauda equina syndromes and neurogenic claudication.

Posterior region of disc is divided into five segments with 20% each, viz: Central, lateral (2 on either side) and far lateral (2 on either side). Central and lateral are within the spinal canal. A line drawn medial to the *pedicles divides* lateral from far-lateral space. Far-lateral space is further divided into foraminal and extraforaminal **(Fig. 1.10)**. At the level of disc the degenerated material can prolapse at any one of the said regions and thus named as central disc, prolapse, lateral disc prolapse, foraminal disc prolapse and extraforaminal disc prolapse. While many of the lateral disc prolapses are symptomatic, those at extraforaminal are asymptomatic at large. Migration of disc materials are common in both directions, viz: superiorly and inferiorly and can either be at lateral or central. Thus migrated disc materials can get lodged in lateral canal below the pedicles or can be seen in nerve root canal toward the foramen exit. Combination of all the types can be seen sometimes. Centrally migrated discs can be seen behind the scalloped posterior vertebral body. Majority of these migrated materials are sequestrated **(Fig. 1.11)**.

Degenerated disc material (nucleus pulposus) when stay-contained within the disc (below annulus) is called contained disc prolapse. It becomes extruded when it transgresse the annulus but still connected to the nucleus inside. Extruded disc material can then get detached separately from nucleus inside and become sequestrated. During this process, the disc material can stay subannulus, below posterior longitudinal ligament or transgress PLL and become extradural totally. Rarely, dura is violated. Intradural disc prolapses are reported but I have not come across the one so far **(Fig. 1.12)**.

Generally, central and lateral disc prolapses can be managed through interlaminar approach. Migrated discs can be removed by extending the bone removal on appropriate direction. In relation to the nerve root, the disc material can be approached either through shoulder or axillary approach whichever provides the easy access **(Fig. 1.13)**.

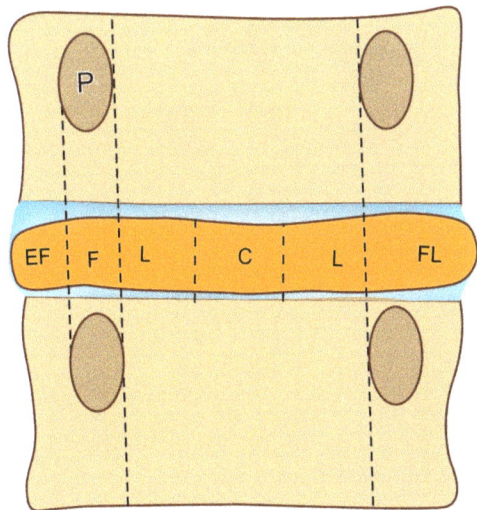

Fig. 1.10 Level of disc space
Abbreviations: C, central; EF, extraforaminal; F, foraminal; FL, far lateral; L, lateral; P, pedicle

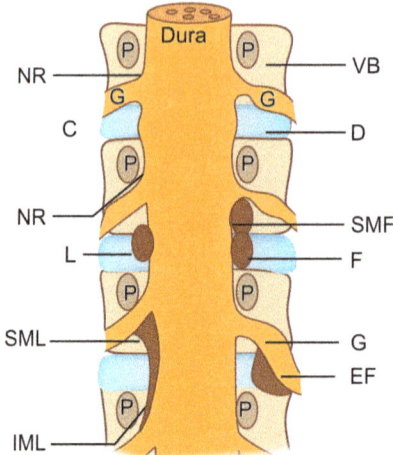

Fig. 1.11 Disc prolapses and sites
Abbreviations: P, pedicle; VB, vertebral body; D, disc; NR, nerve root; G, ganglion; C, central disc prolapse; L, lateral disc prolapse; F, foraminal disc prolapse; SMF, superior migrated foraminal; EF, extraforaminal; SML, superior migrated lateral; IML, inferior migrated lateral

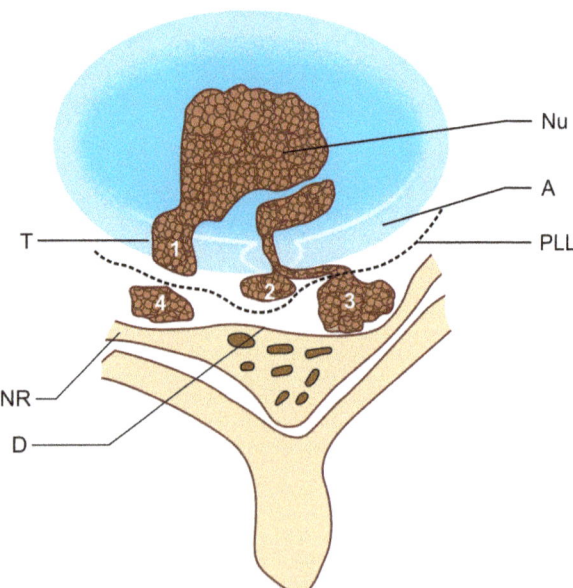

Fig. 1.12 Disc prolapse; 1. Subannular disc prolapse (contained), 2. Extruded sub PLL disc prolapse, 3. Extruded extradural disc prolapse, 4. Sequestrated disc prolapse
Abbreviations: Nu, nucleus pulposus; A, annulus; T, Tear (rent); PLL, posterior longitudinal ligament; NR, nerve root; D, dural sac ventral

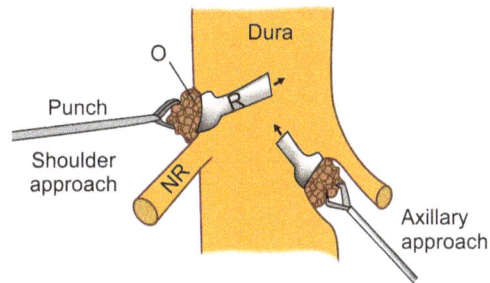

Fig. 1.13 Approach in relation to nerve root
Abbreviations: R, nerve root retractor; NR, nerve root; O, disc

Foraminal, some superiorly migrated and extraforaminal disc prolapses can be managed through far-lateral and transforaminal approaches. The details of the techniques are given in subsequent chapters.

CHAPTER 2

Preoperative Preparations

POSITIONING

After endotracheal intubation, the patient is positioned prone over two bolsters that are tied together with adequate gap between each other depending on the patient's body width **(Figs 2.1A to E)**. Bolsters support the lateral aspect of the body, viz. lateral aspect of clavicle and shoulder, lateral aspect of chest and iliac crest thus leaving the mid-portion of chest and abdomen free between the two, bolsters. Free abdomen is essential for good controlled ventilation. Bolsters are firm and made up of rolled rubber cushion covered by good quality leather. The patient is positioned in such a way that the level of surgery is placed over the table where the plates can be bent thus flexing the lumbar spine. This bending improves widening of the interlaminar space and can be easily done in thin, tall patients with flat and moderately

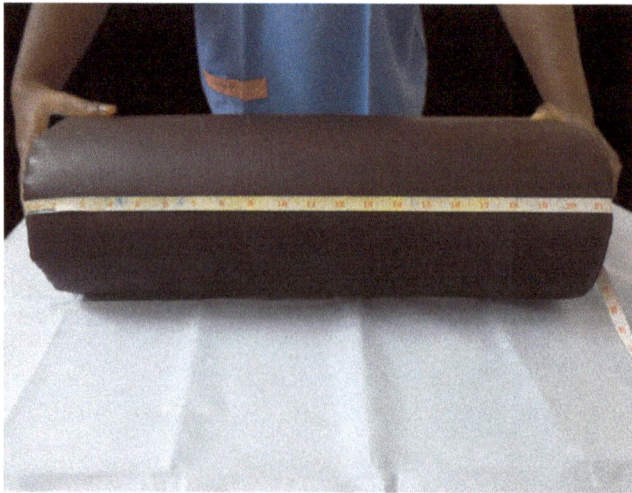

Fig. 2.1A Leather bolster

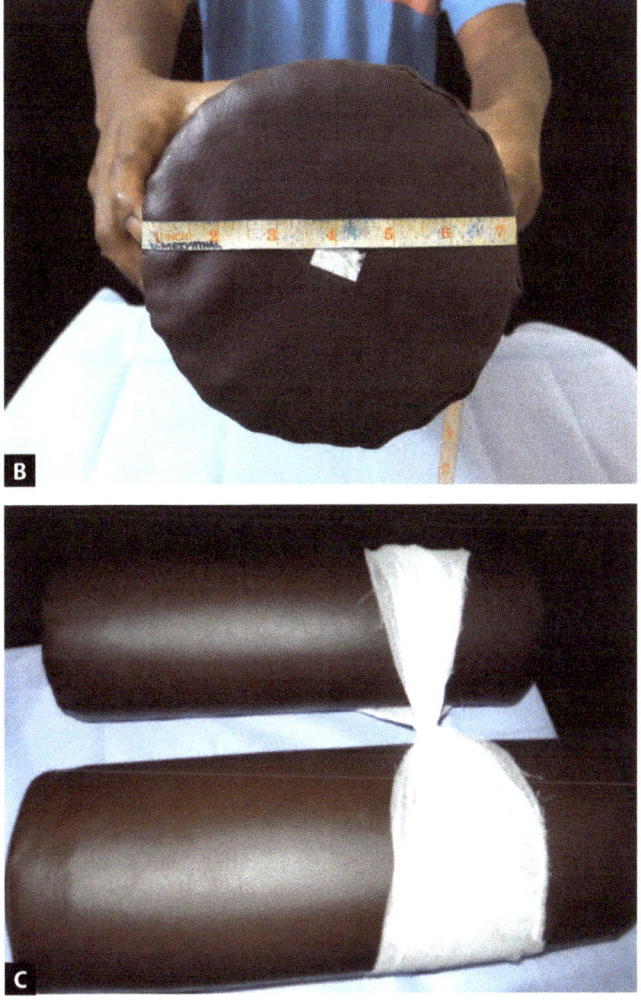

Figs 2.1B and C (B) Diameter of bolster; (C) Two bolsters tied together

obese patients. The jack knife can be achieved to the maximum until satisfactory free abdomen between the bolsters is confirmed. In case the abdomen is not free, it is better to reduce flexion. A free abdomen is essential for two reasons: to secure good respiration and to avoid congestion of Batson's plexus and hence prevent uncomfortable epidural bleeding during the procedure **(Fig. 2.2)**.

Appropriate sized bolsters should be selected for different patients. Very long bolsters will cause compression over side of neck and femoral nerve and vessel compression. Sometimes, cotton sheet supports can be placed below

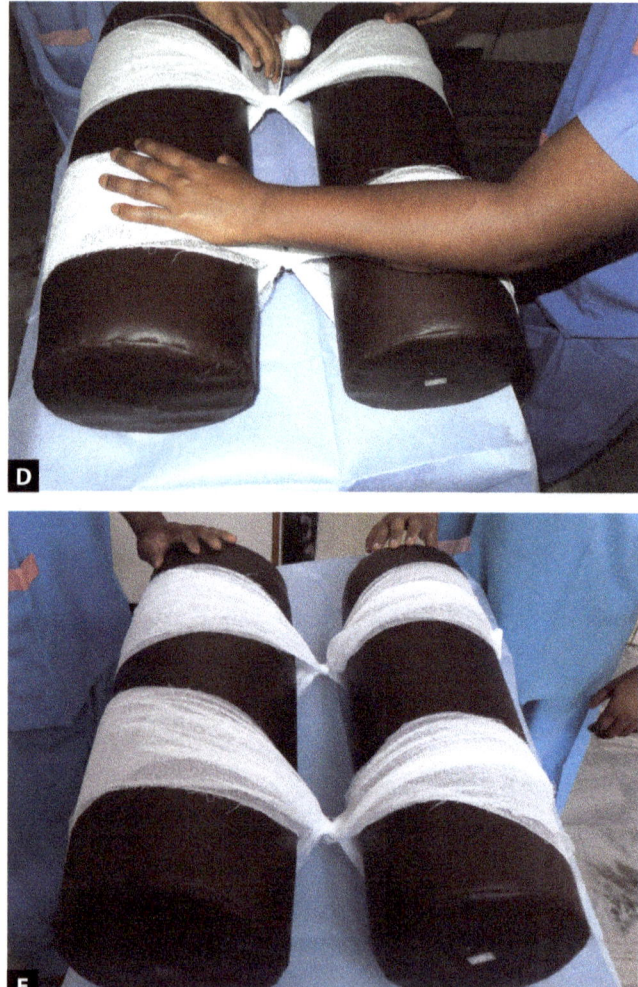

Figs 2.1D and E Method of preparing the bolsters

the iliac crest to prevent femoral region compression. Longer bolsters hinder the security of endotracheal tube and the face, are seen hidden between the bolsters, which is not acceptable. Very short bolsters will fail to support the hip and hence dangerous for the femorals.

Various sizes of bolsters should be available in the theater to suit different sized patients. Standard bolsters are 20″ in length with 2″ in addition and 6″ in diameter. Different length bolster 20″, 22″, 24″and 26″ should be available. We do have bolsters with 8″ in diameter for heavy patients without large protruding abdomen. In extraordinary patients with lax and protruding abdomen, we avoid bolsters and use the chest pelvis pillows.

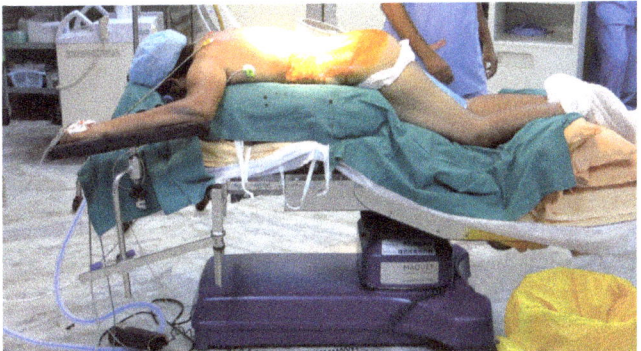

Fig. 2.2 Prone position—patient placed on the bolsters

In all patients, the knee should be flexed and shin and ankle supported well. The neck should be straight and face, eyes protected with eye guards and head placed over a horseshoe cushion rest. The endotracheal tube should be free, accessible and secured at all time. The upper limbs are supported by hand rest with good cushions at joints and placed on head-end side.

For MLD catheterization of bladder is still controversial. However, in my practice-I catheterize all my patients with indwelling urinary catheter and remove them in postoperative period. This is to just avoid bladder distension during surgery since the patients are on intravenous fluids during surgery. A free bladder prevents intra-abdominal pressure, which is essential for a docile Batson's plexus. If one encounters uncomfortable epidural bleed due to bladder distension during the procedure, then my view of catheterizing the patient will be accepted without much controversy. Catheter must be carefully placed between the bolsters and always check the penis for confirmation of no compression.

LEVEL MARKING

Marking the level of correct disc space is important in MLD. Since the incision is small, one needs to be accurate in marking the level of interest. In prone position and when lumbar spine is well-flexed, the tip of upper spinous process corresponds to disc level. For example, L_4 spinous process tip corresponds to L_4/L_5 disc space. In thin individuals it is easy to mark since the thickness of skin and its subcutaneous is relatively thin. However, anatomical correlation between spinous process and disc space may not be correct in fat, large and in patients with huge body mass. The distance between skin and spinous process is crucial. When a patient is well-flexed at lumbar region this is reduced due to the stretching of skin and subcutaneous tissues. Hence, when a patient is placed without flexion and placed straight (neutral) over the bolsters, then not only we observe increase in distance between skin and spinous process but also crowding of spinous processes.

This is often noticed in very bulky individuals. Hence, level marking becomes an art for a perfect surgery to begin.

After placing the patient in position, insert a small but thick needle just below the spinous process of L_4 for L_4/L_5 disc level and take a lateral view X-ray using image intensifier and confirm the site **(Fig. 2.3)**. If not satisfactory reinsert the needle accordingly until you get the right level. In bulky individual one has to be careful in marking and an imaginary line of dissection should be planned. Occasionally, though the marking may be correct, dissection of paraspinal muscle may be oblique and hence reach the wrong level. Hence, it is always better to recheck with image intensifier after or during dissection when in doubt. Never proceed when in doubt and no need to worry for recheck. This step will help you in achieving zero percent wrong level in your practice.

A word of caution in level marking: It is surgeon's responsibility to mark them correctly. It is my practice to read the scans and X-rays myself and correlate them with image intensifier at the time of marking and I never go with radiological reports, which may misguide since the reading and understanding of lumbosacral region especially in sacralization of lumbar spine and anatomical variations may vary between clinicians. Surgeons should never blame others for wrong level exploration. Hence, read the radiological investigations yourself and mark the level.

The needle site is marked horizontally either with a sterile marker pen or a needle on the skin and 25 mm vertical line is marked just lateral to the midline on the side of exposure with needle site as midpoint.

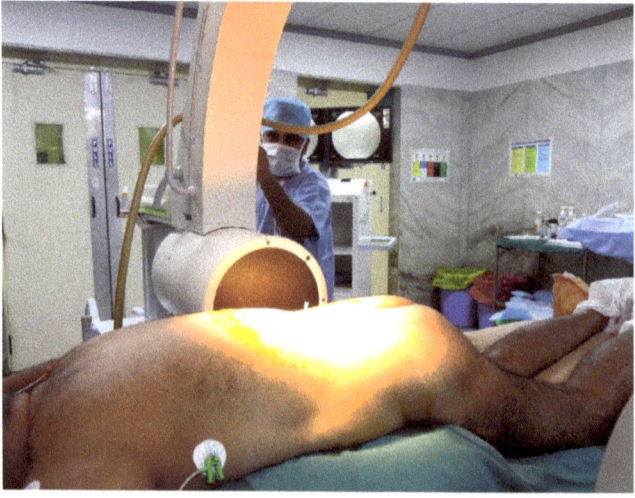

Fig. 2.3 Marking the site with image intensifier guidance

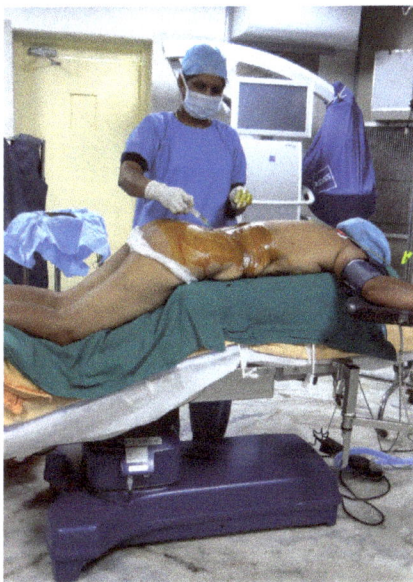

Fig. 2.4 Operative site prepared

PREPARATION OF OPERATING SITE

The skin over the operating site is prepared well with aseptic precautions. Skin is prepared with povidone iodine scrub (10%) and chlorhexidine gluconate and alcohol solution. Subcutaneous tissue is injected with 5 mL of 2% lignocaine. Now the site is painted with 5% povidone iodine solution and draped exposing the skin mark for incision **(Fig. 2.4)**.

CHAPTER 3

Operative Techniques with Case Examples

INTERLAMINAR APPROACH

Lateral Disc Prolapse—Lower Level

Case example: Small lateral disc prolapse in a spacious spinal canal with nerve root compression on the right side.

Clinical status: Sciatica right leg **(Figs 3.1A and 1B)**.

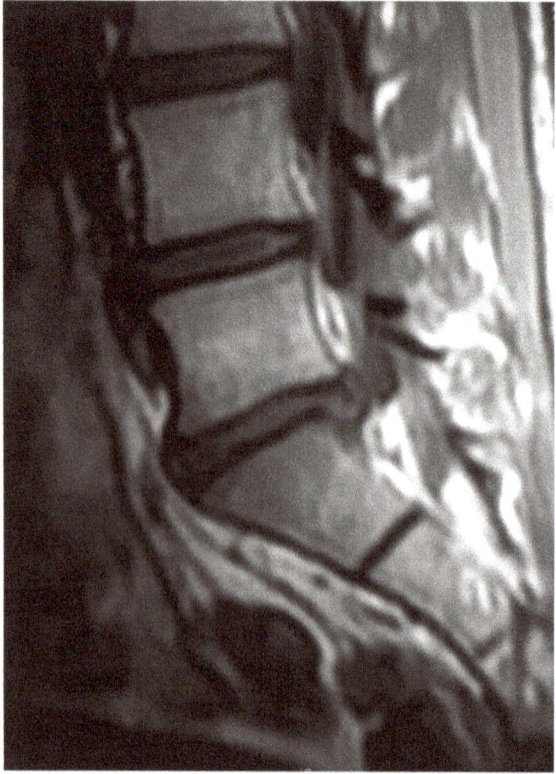

Fig. 3.1A: MRI sagittal view showing L_5/S_1 small disc prolapse

Operative Techniques with Case Examples

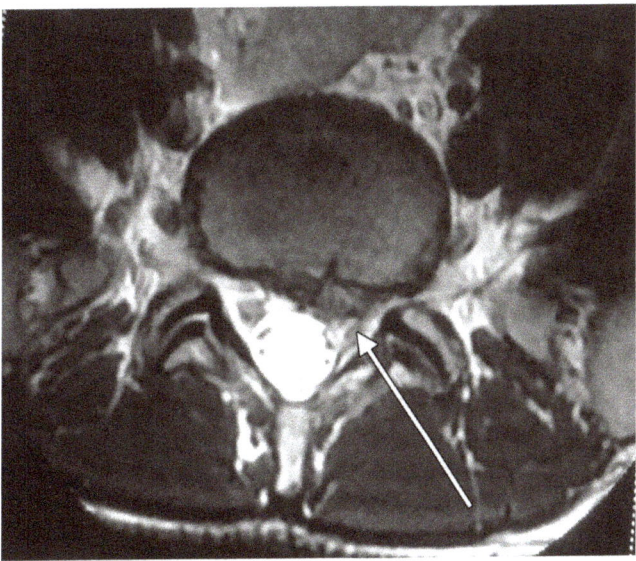

Fig. 3.1B: MRI axial view showing lateral disc prolapse with nerve root compression

Operative Procedure (Fig. 3.2)

Step 1–Incision: Skin is incised in the midline over the upper spinous process to an approximate length of 25 mm using a sharp surgical knife **(Figs 3.3 and 3.4)**. The subcutaneous layer is entered and loose areolar tissue with fat and cut blood vessels encountered. Haemostasis is achieved with bipolar cautery **(Fig. 3.5)**. Skin and subcutaneous layer is then retracted with a small two- or three-prong retractor and surgical wound is widened **(Figs 3.6 to 3.9)**.

Step 2–Exposure of interlaminar space: The dorsolumbar fascia is cut just lateral to the spinous process to the entire length or more under the skin towards both ends **(Figs 3.10 to 3.12)**. This exposes the paraspinal muscle

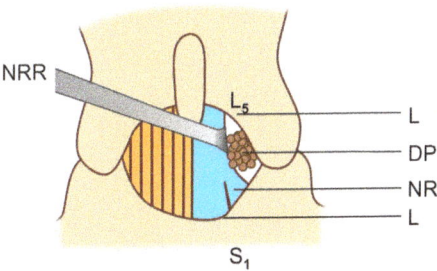

Fig. 3.2
Abbreviations: DP, Disc prolapse; L, lamina; NR, nerve root; NRR, nerve root retractor

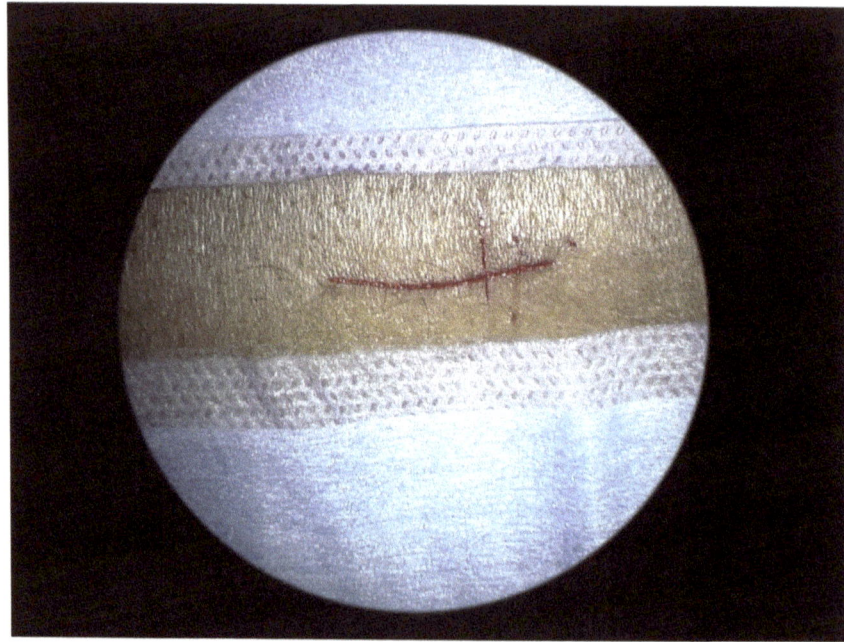

Fig. 3.3: Skin marking

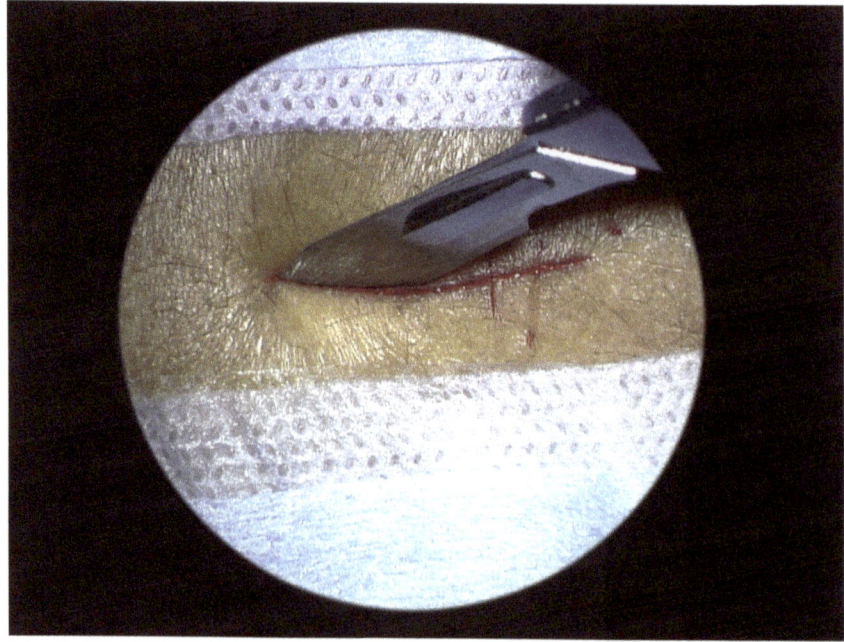

Fig. 3.4: Skin incision with No. 10 surgical blade

Operative Techniques with Case Examples | 19

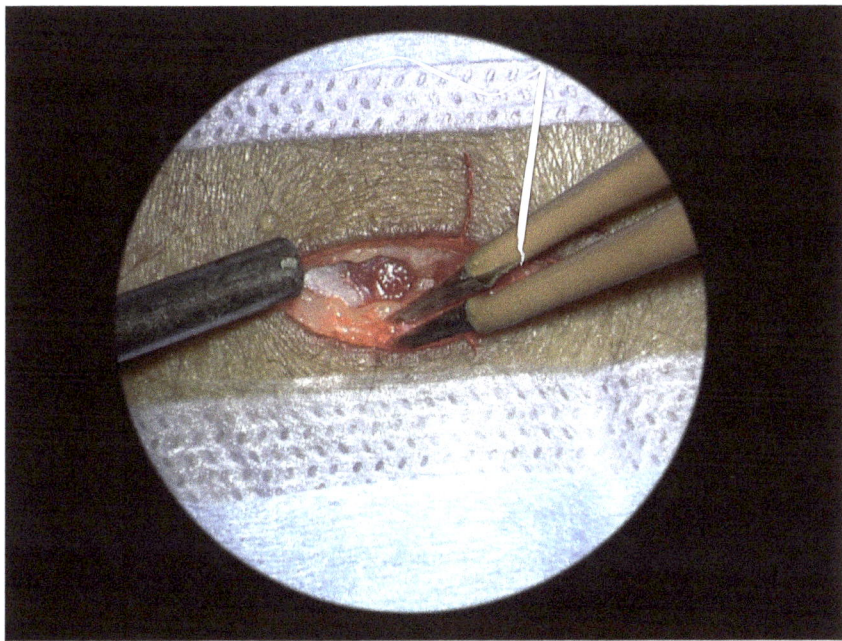

Fig. 3.5: Bipolar cautery of subcutaneous bleeders

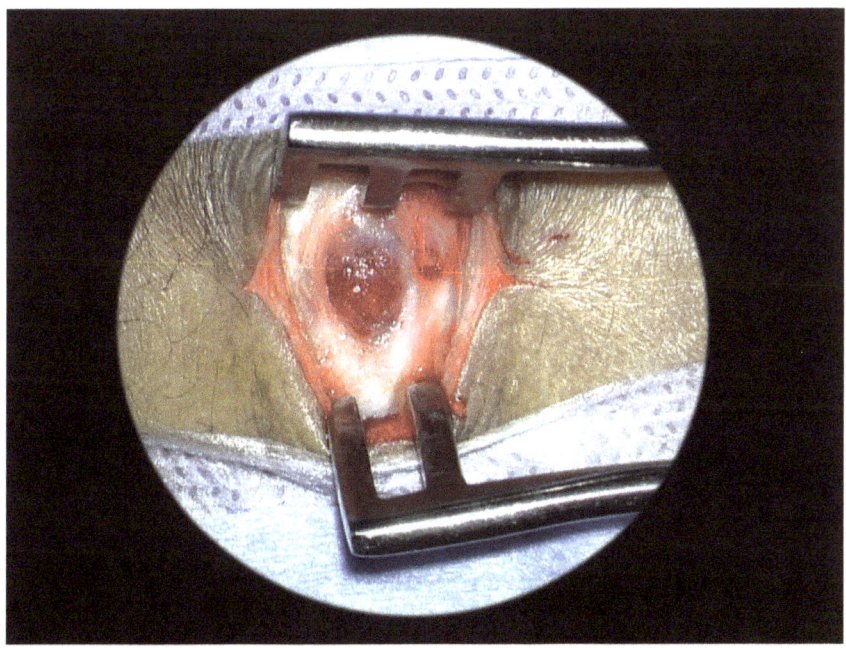

Fig. 3.6: Skin retracted with double (or) triple pronged retractor

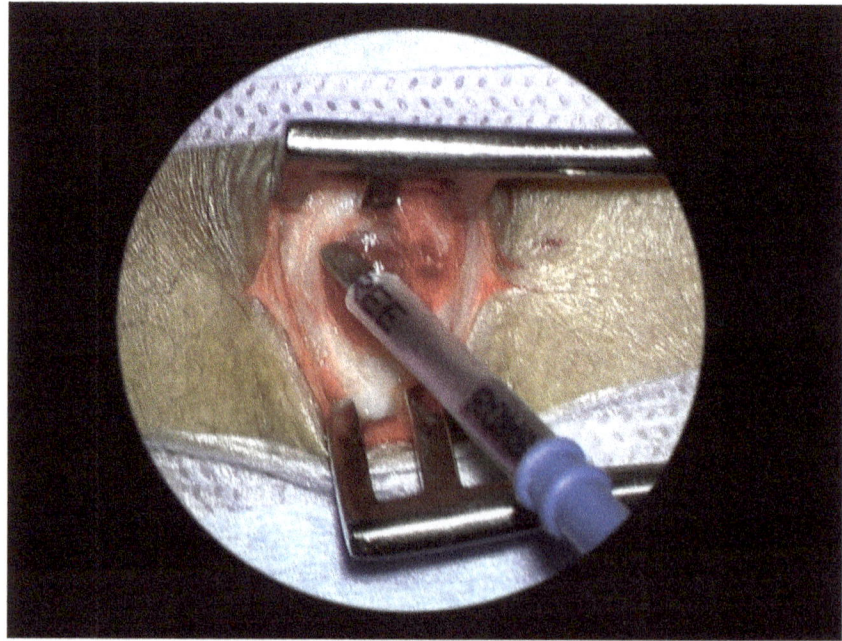

Fig. 3.7: Monopolar cautery cuts the soft tissues

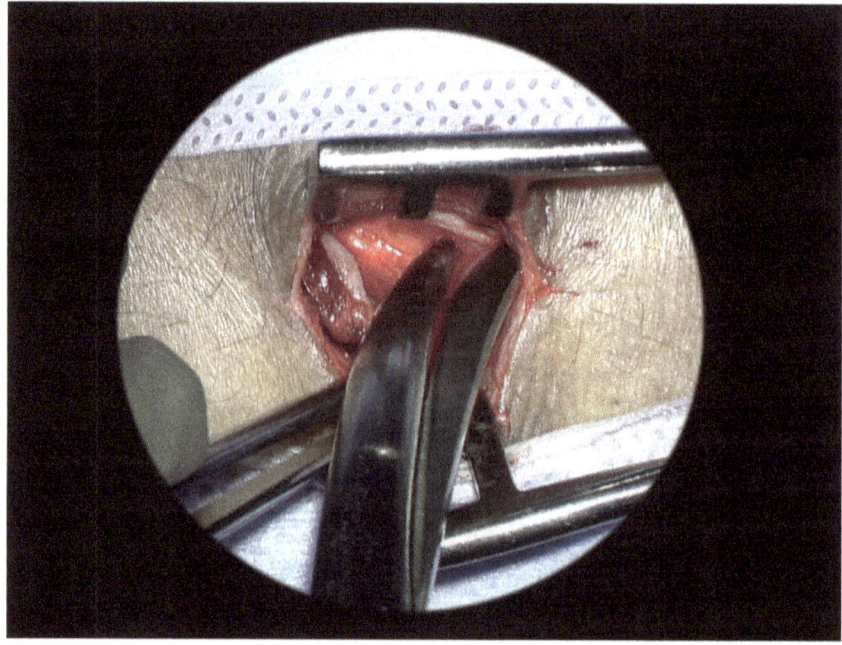

Fig. 3.8: Further dissection done with blunt scissors

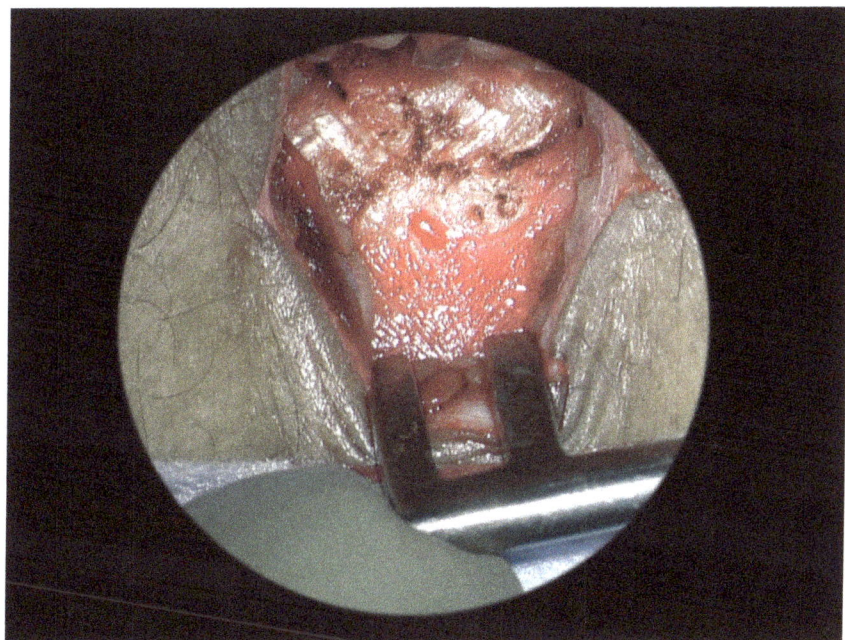

Fig. 3.9: Retractor blades reapplied to expose dorsolumbar fascia

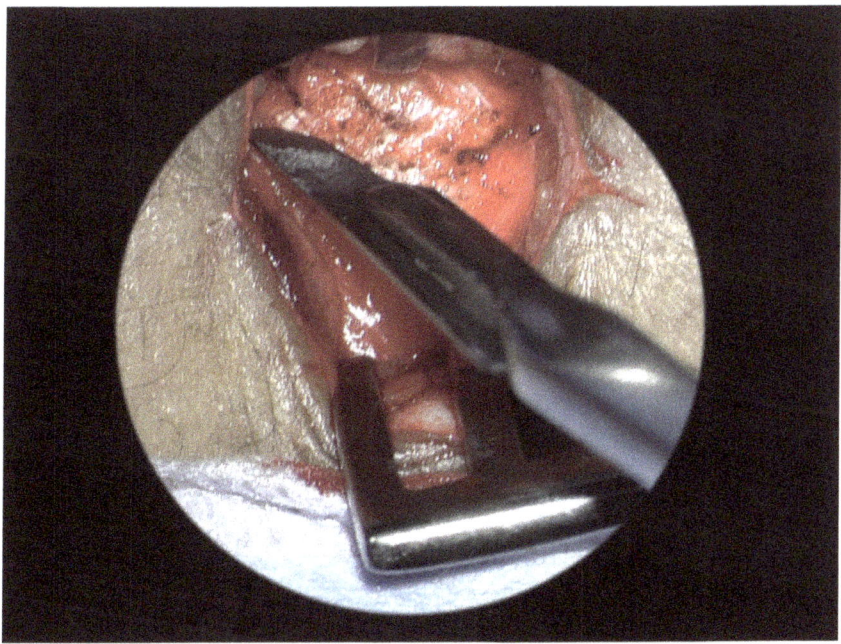

Fig. 3.10: Dorsolumbar fascia is cut in the midline using No. 15 surgical knife

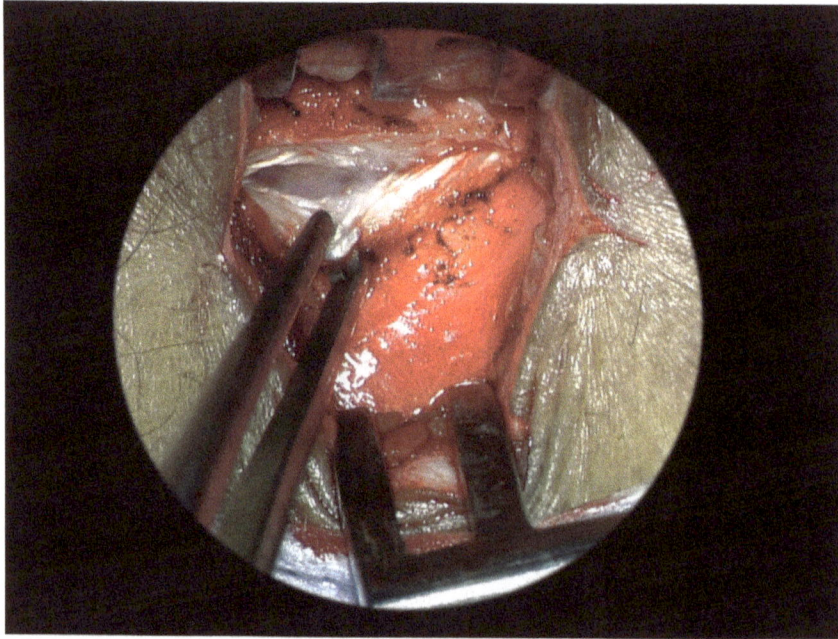

Fig. 3.11: Fascia lifted with a tooth forceps

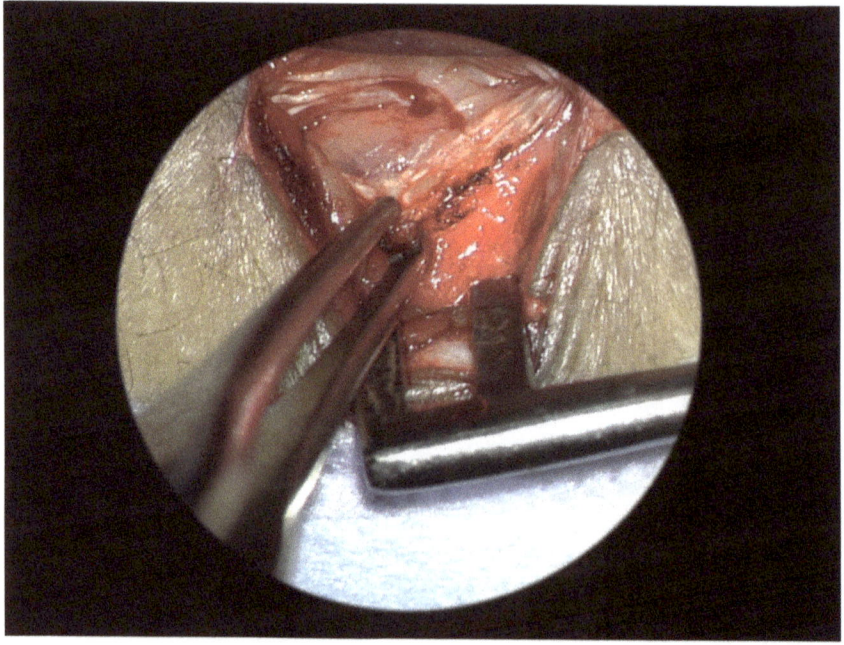

Fig. 3.12: Fascia is cut liberally just lateral to the spinous process

which is then retracted laterally and subperiosteal dissection is made with low cautery and stripped over the sides of spinous process and lamina of superior vertebra **(Figs 3.13 and 3.14)**. The muscle is further retracted from inferior lamina too. Low cautery dissection is very effective in maintaining a bloodless field all along. When the muscle is retracted with a Langenbergh retractor, following structures are exposed: Interlaminar space filled with soft tissues and lateral surface of spinous process. Laminar surface of adjacent spine and medial surface of facet joint **(Figs 3.15 to 3.16)**. Soft tissue in the interlaminar space like fat and tissues need to be removed to expose ligamentum flavum **(Fig. 3.17)**. Now double-hook retractor blades are positioned to retract the muscle until the procedure is over **(Figs 3.18 to 3.25)**.

Step 3–Exposure of epidual region: Ligamentum flavum is tough and stretched due to postioning. Using a number 12 knife, the ligament is cut across from medial to lateral layer by layer with out-exerting pressure **(Fig. 3.26)**. When outer layers are cut, one can appreciate retracting fibers thus providing better vision at depth **(Fig. 3.27)**. Gentle stroke of cut over deepest fibers exposes epidural fat and sometimes dural sleeves are very close. Once ligamentum flavum is cut, it can be removed with Kerrison punches **(Figs 3.28 and 3.29)**. Care should be taken when ligament is thick and buckled. Usually a well-flexed lumbar spine keeps the ligamentum stretched and hence easy

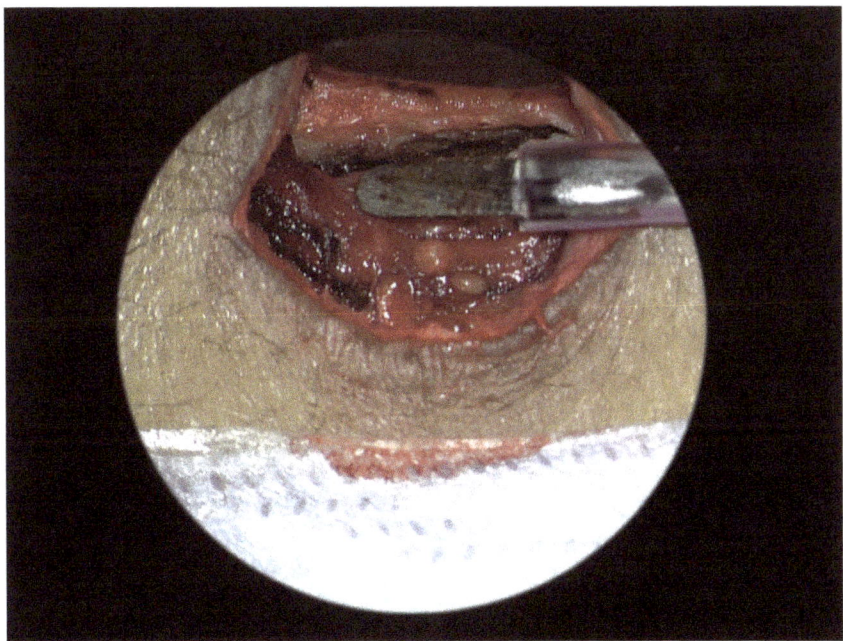

Fig. 3.13: Monopolar cautery used to mobilize paraspinal muscle subperiosteally

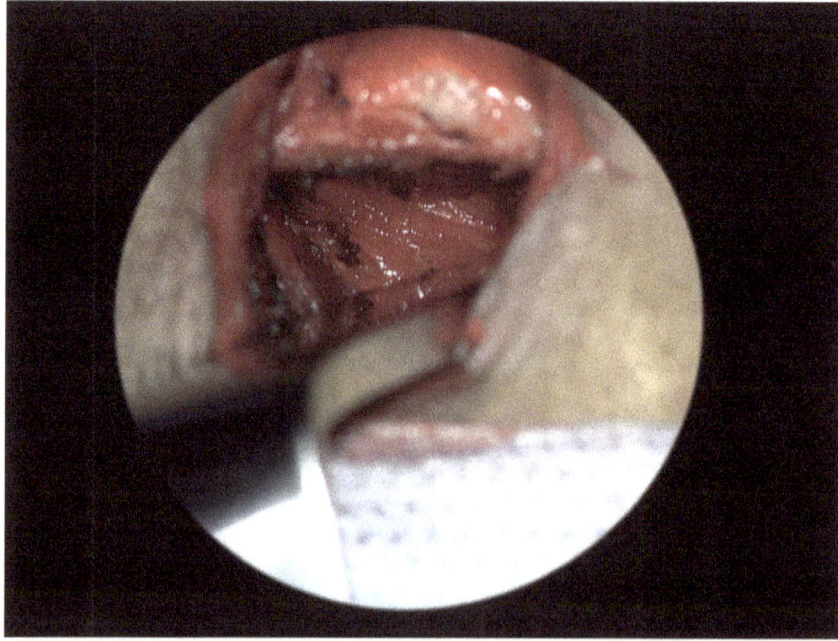

Fig. 3.14: Paraspinal muscle thus detached is retracted well

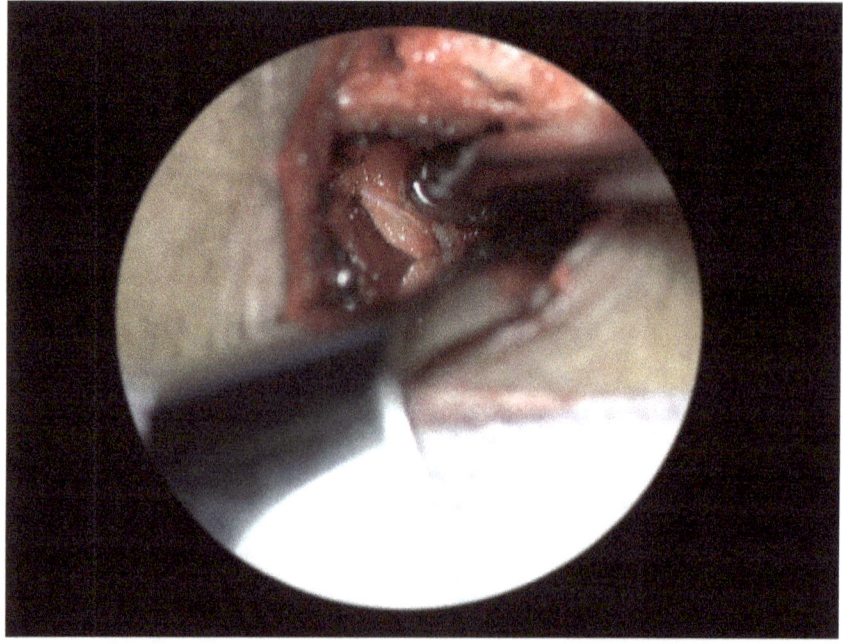

Fig. 3.15: Soft tissue under the muscle and in the interlaminar space are removed with a tissue forceps

Operative Techniques with Case Examples | 25

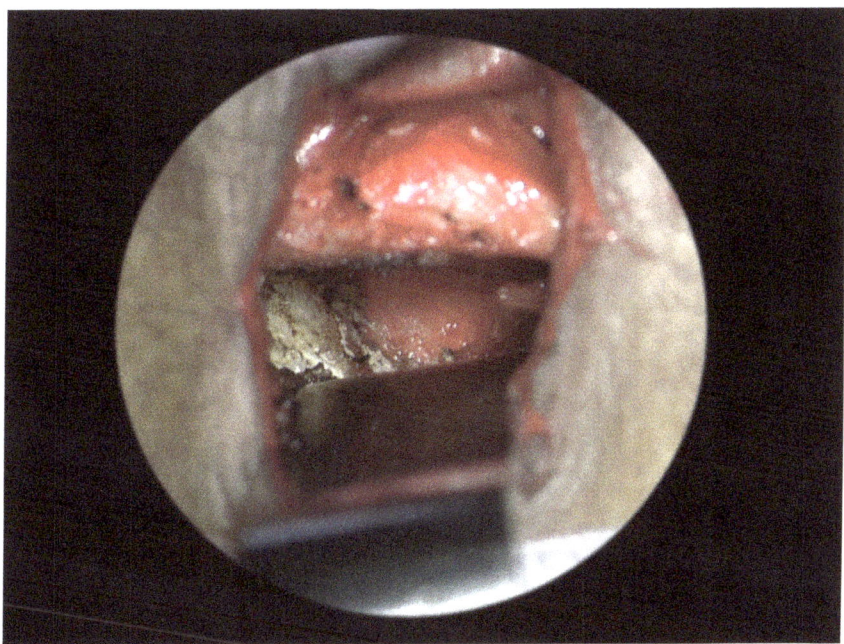

Fig. 3.16: Lamina and interlaminar space well defined

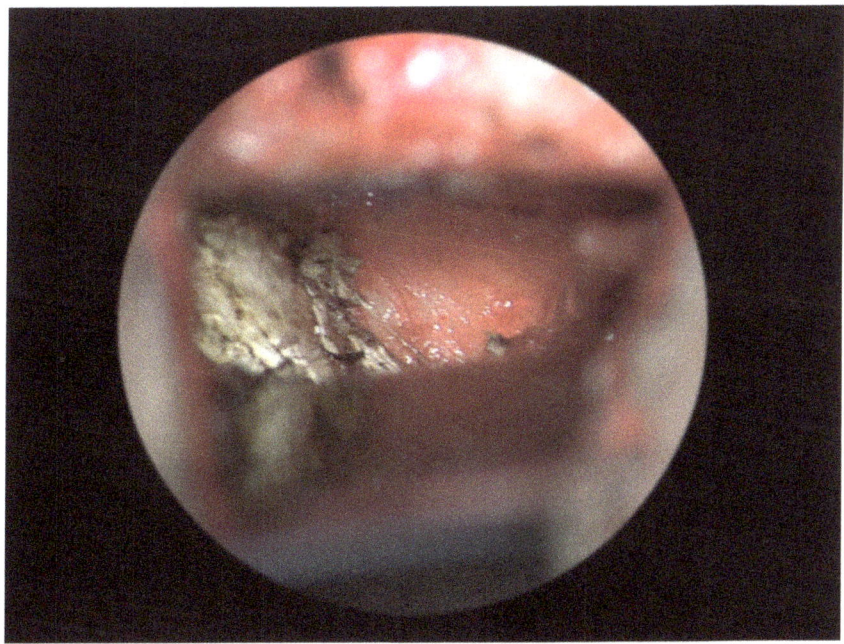

Fig. 3.17: Ligamentum flavum exposed. Magnification of view is further increased

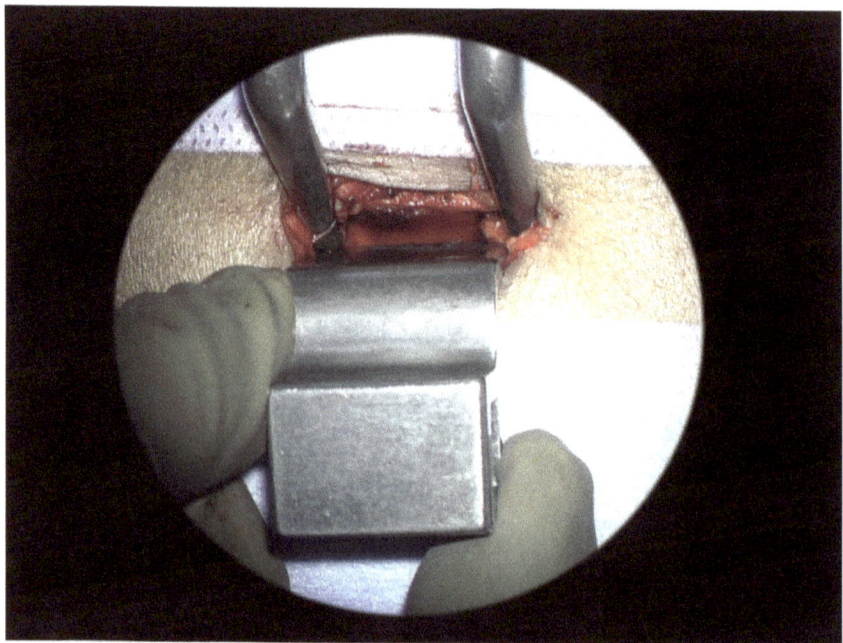

Fig. 3.18: Micro lumbar double hook retractor is introduced. Hooks over the spinous process

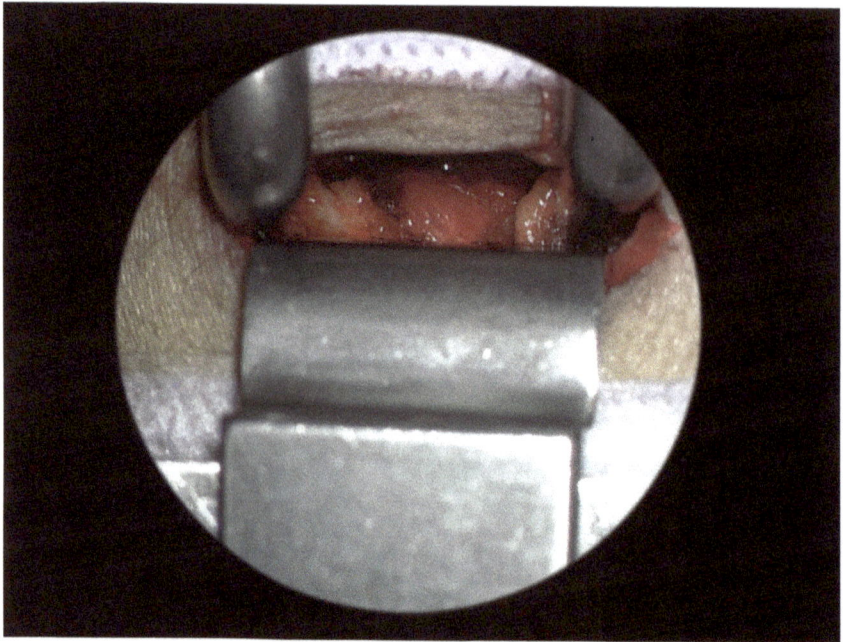

Fig. 3.19: Flat blade retracts the paraspinal muscle

Operative Techniques with Case Examples | 27

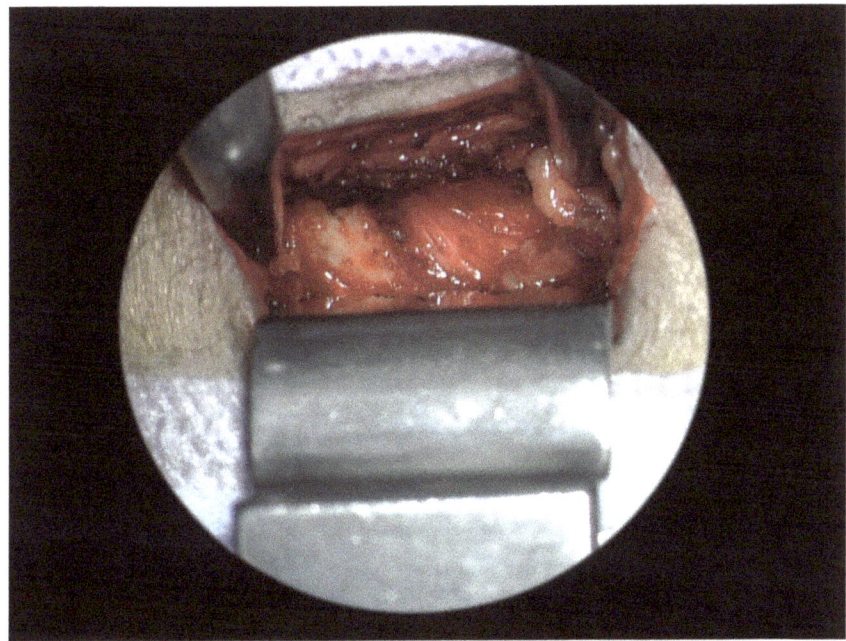

Fig. 3.20: Blades are retracted. Hooks rest over the spinous process and the muscle retracted against the bone

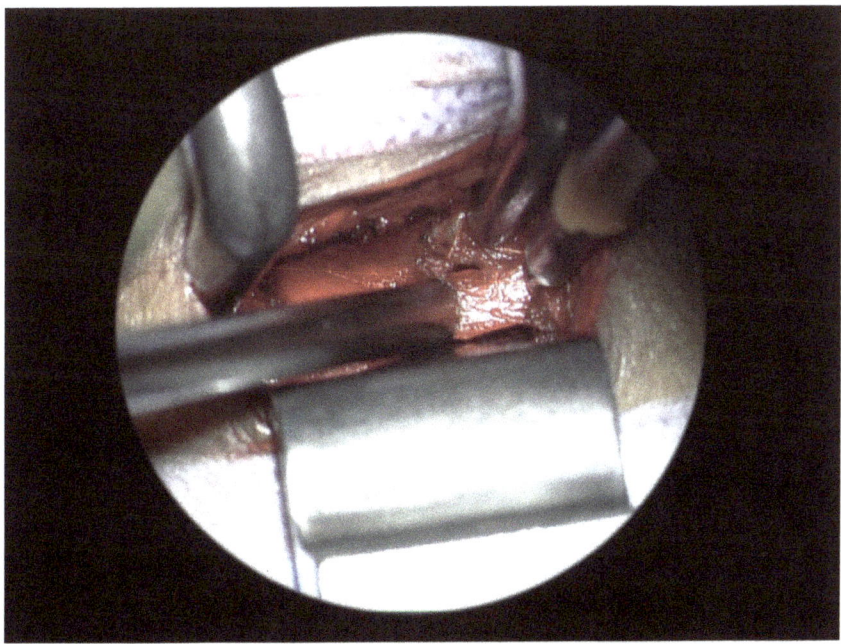

Fig. 3.21: Protruding soft tissues are removed

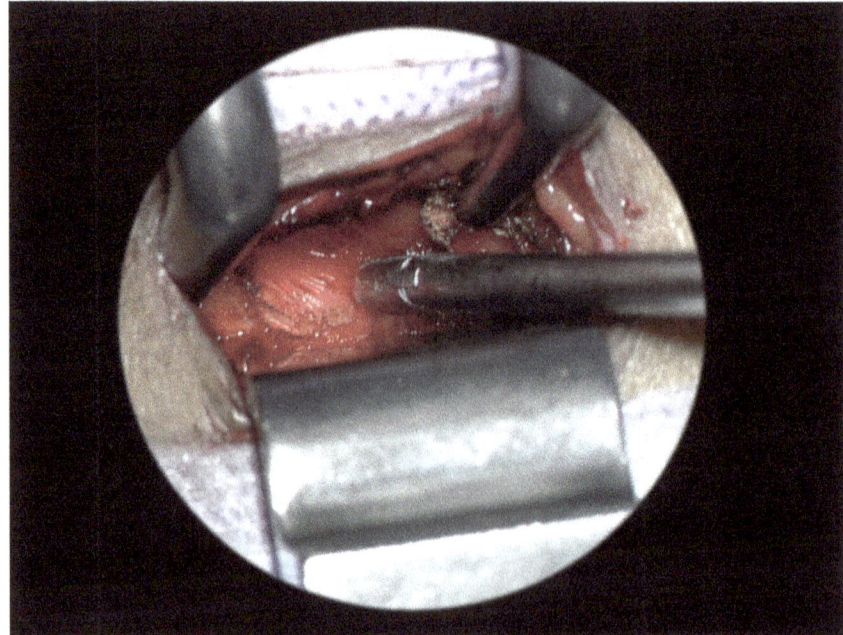

Fig. 3.22: Further soft tissues are removed to get a clear view

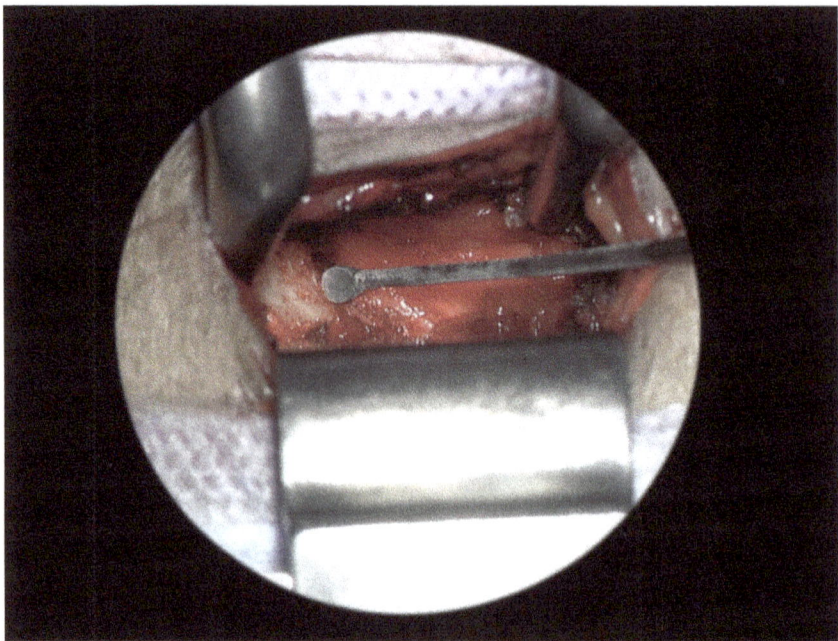

Fig. 3.23: Lower border of upper lamina

Operative Techniques with Case Examples | 29

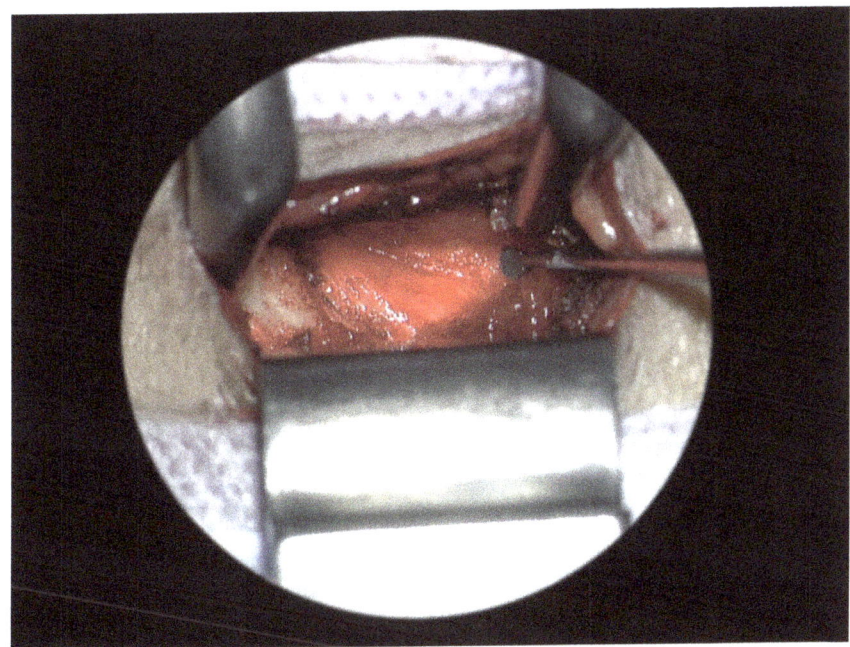

Fig. 3.24: Upper border of lower lamina

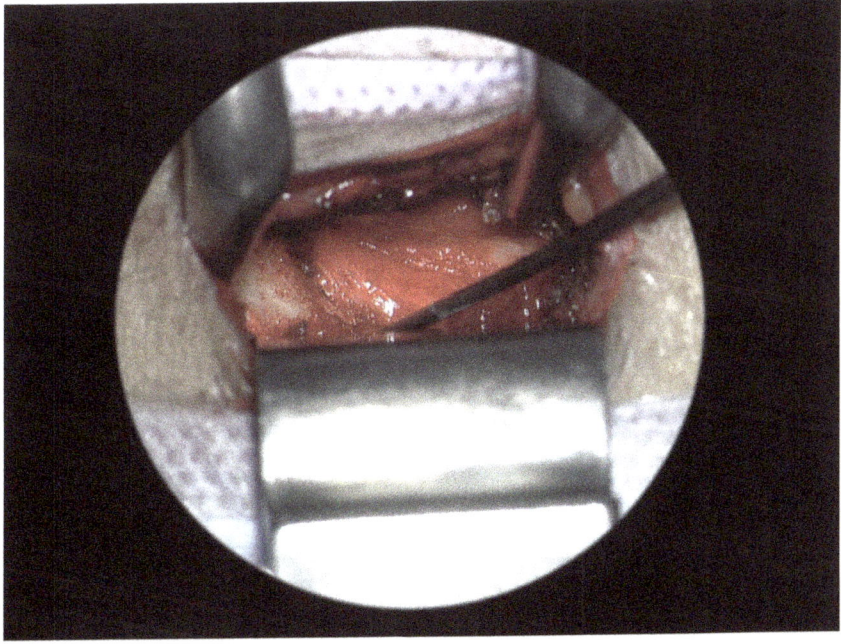

Fig. 3.25: Pointer towards the facet joint laterally

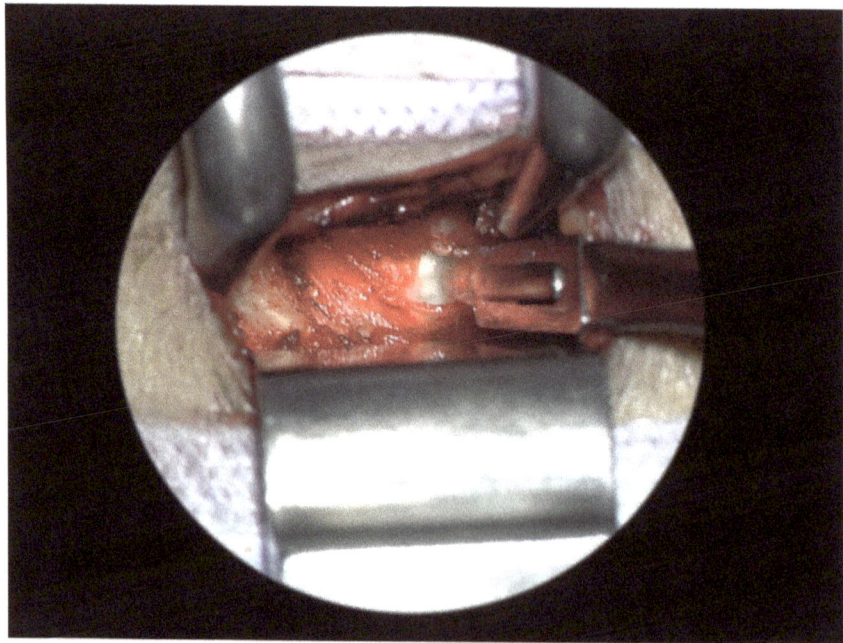

Fig. 3.26: Incise the ligamentum flavum with No. 15 surgical knife just above the upper border of lower lamina

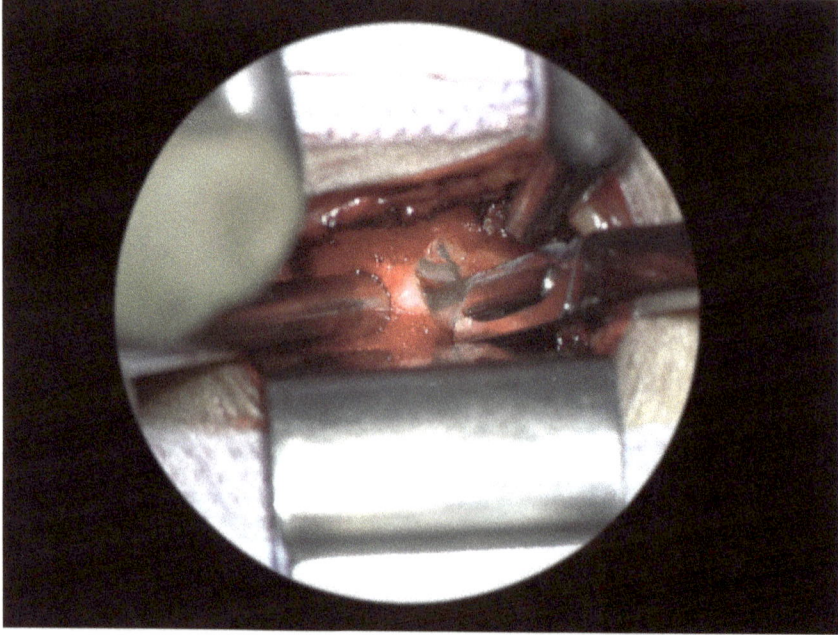

Fig. 3.27: Incision should be deepened layer by layer until the epidural space is visualized

Operative Techniques with Case Examples | 31

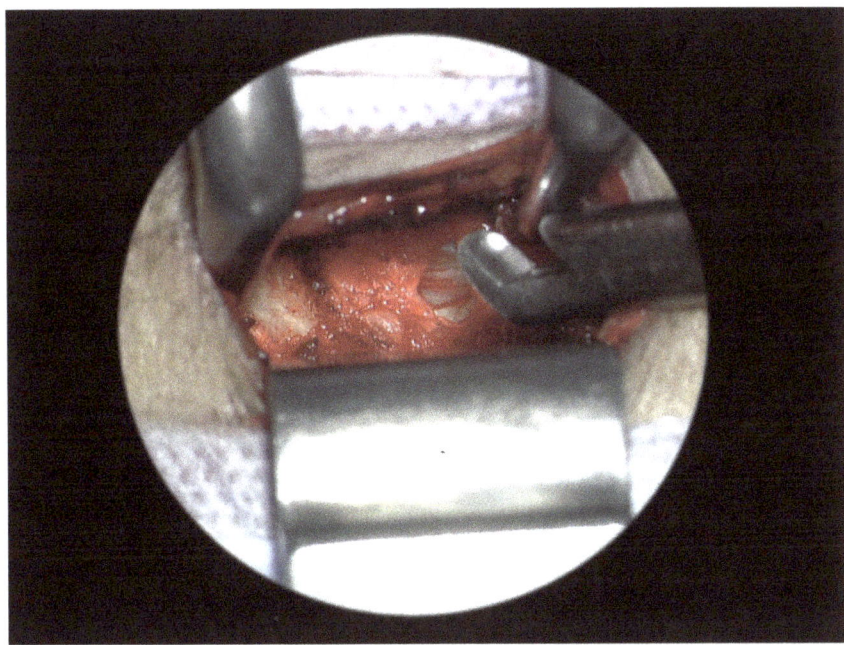

Fig. 3.28: Kerrison punches with 45° angle are ideal choices for excising the ligament

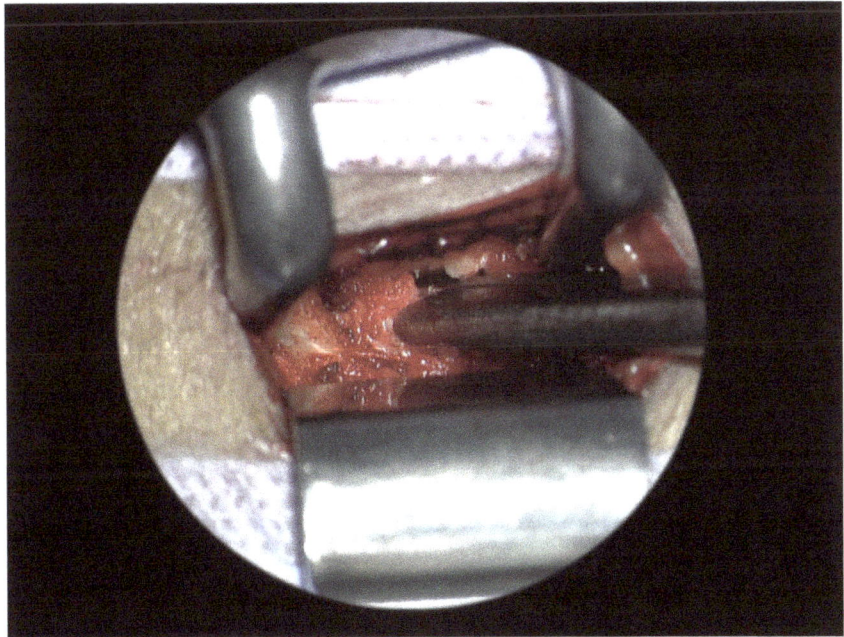

Fig. 3.29: Ligament should be excised meticulously without pressure over underlying structures

to excise. Ligament at the inferior aspect of upper lamina and below the facets should be removed well **(Figs 3.30 and 3.31)**. This will give wider exposure to lateral one third of the disc. In this way, the epidural space in the interlaminar region is exposed liberally **(Fig. 3.32)**.

Step 4-Delineating the nerve root: Epidural space is inspected well and the fat needs to be dissected from superior to inferior and lateral to medial directions. Epidural fat is essential and must be preserved at maximum. Epidural vessels that are part of Batson's plexus should be dissected, cauterized with sharp end bipolar low cautery and cut with sharp microscissors **(Figs 3.33 to 3.35)**. While doing these steps, the surgeon will get a clear idea about dura, nerve root and disc prolapse. Hence while cauterizing the vessels, they need to be picked away from dural sleeve. Once nerve root is identified, its entire length should be inspected carefully **(Fig. 3.36)**. The nerve root is often stretched over underlying bulging annulus or extruded disc material. The dural sleeve is very thin laterally and sometimes difficult to differentiate with annulus. Hence using a small rasperator the nerve root dural sleeve is dissected from structures below from lateral to medial direction. In this way, nerve root can be dissected and retracted medially **(Fig. 3.37)**. Overstretching should be avoided at all cost.

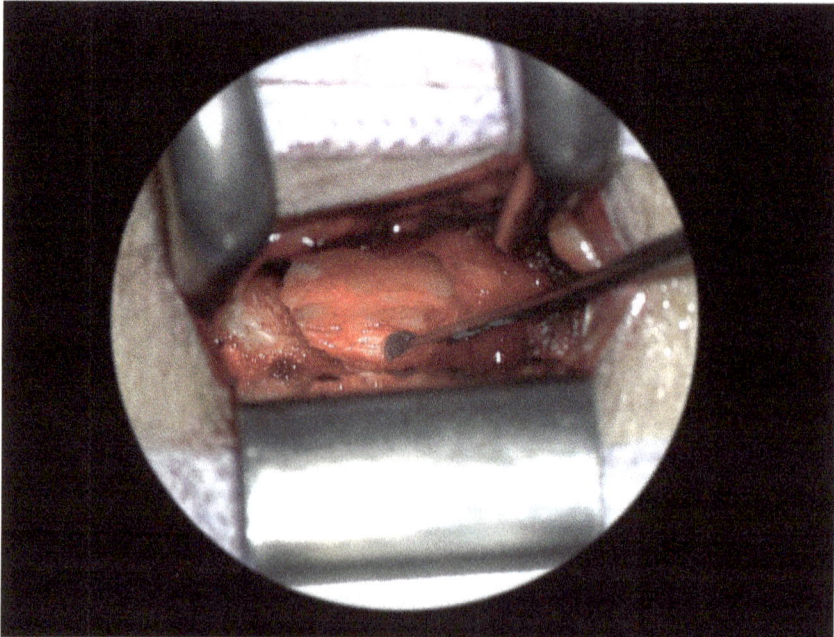

Fig. 3.30: The lateral part of the ligament is very important and that need to be excised to view the lateral border of nerve root and also the lateral 1/3rd of disc

Operative Techniques with Case Examples | 33

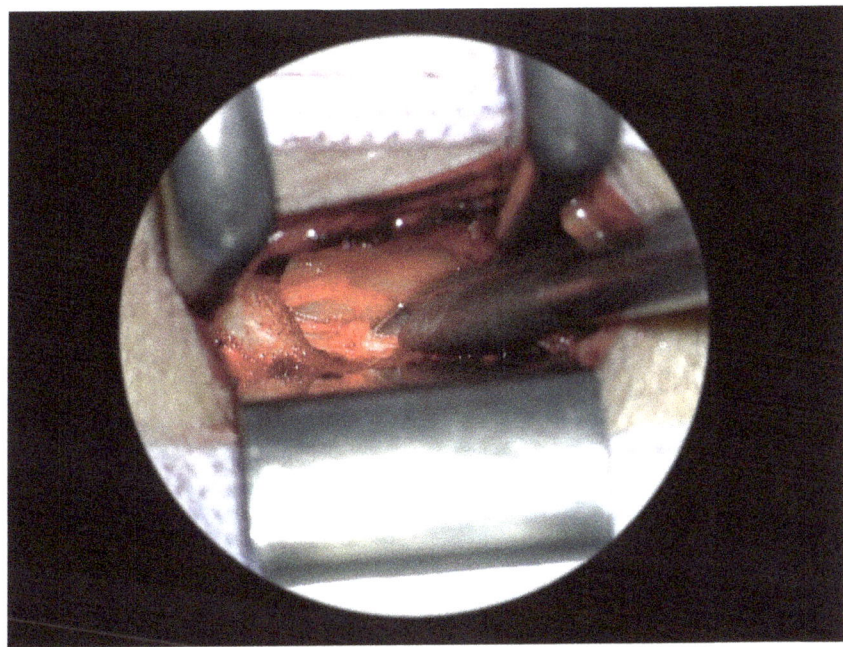

Fig. 3.31: Meticulous removal of lateral part of ligament

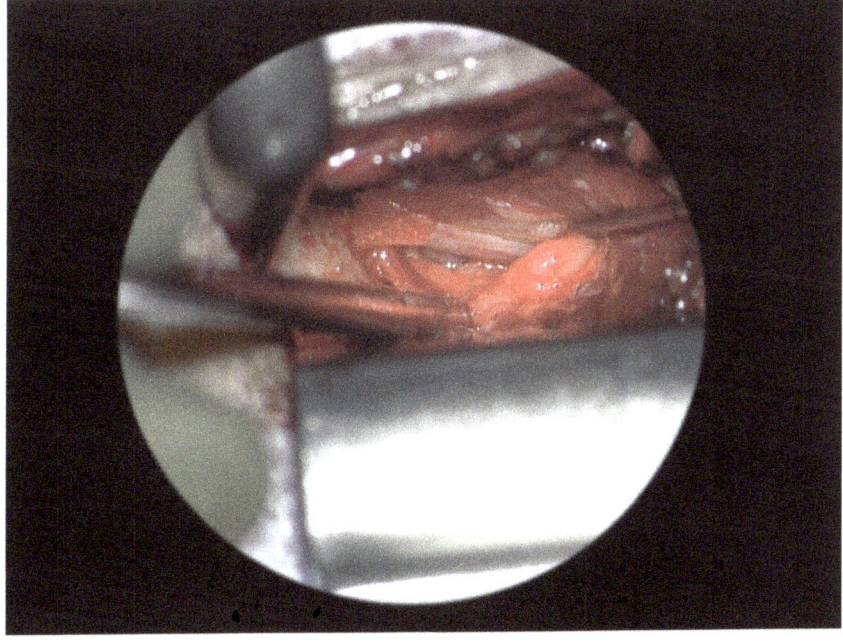

Fig. 3.32: Dissect fat gently to expose the nerve root

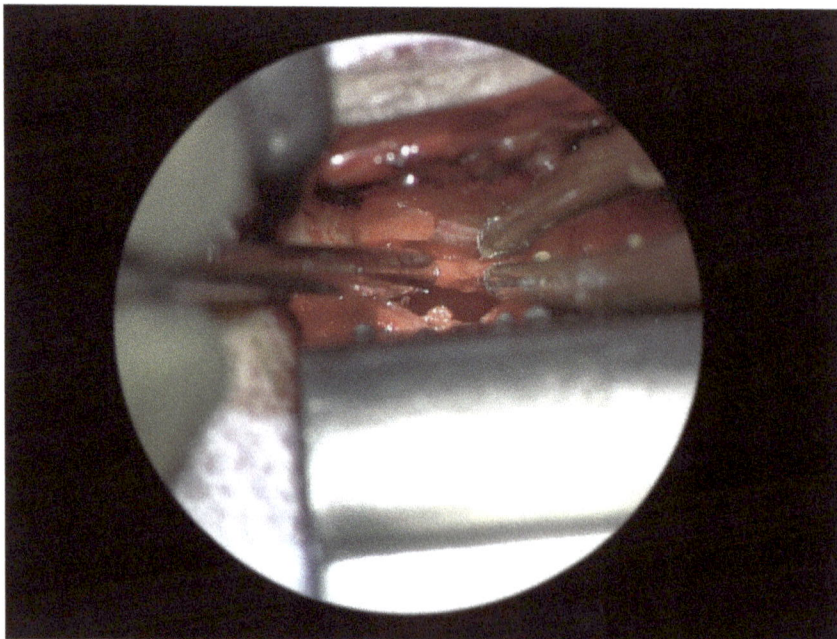

Fig. 3.33: Fat lobules can be shrunk with bipolar cautery to get better visibility

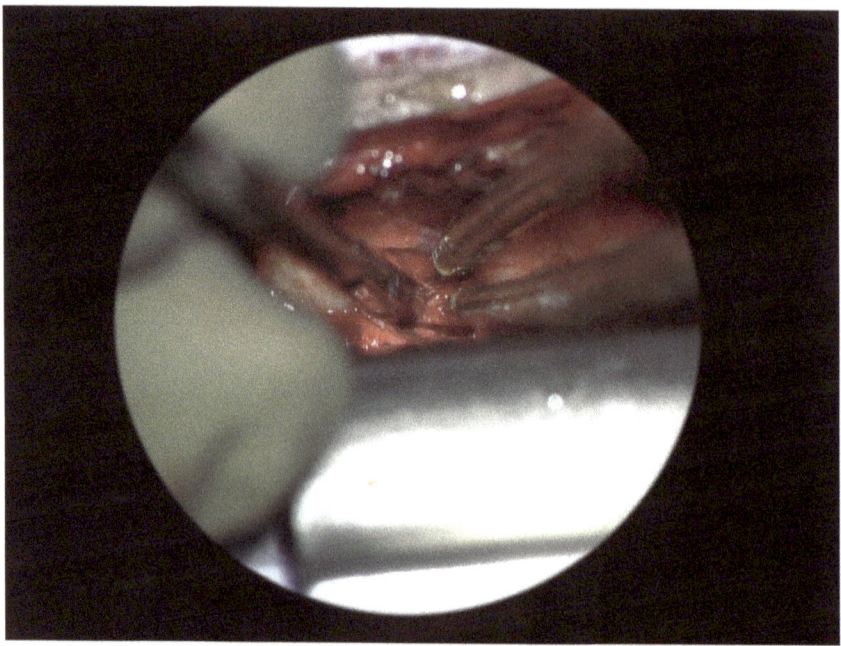

Fig. 3.34: Epidural bleeders and small vessels need to be coagulated with micro-tip bipolar cautery

Operative Techniques with Case Examples | 35

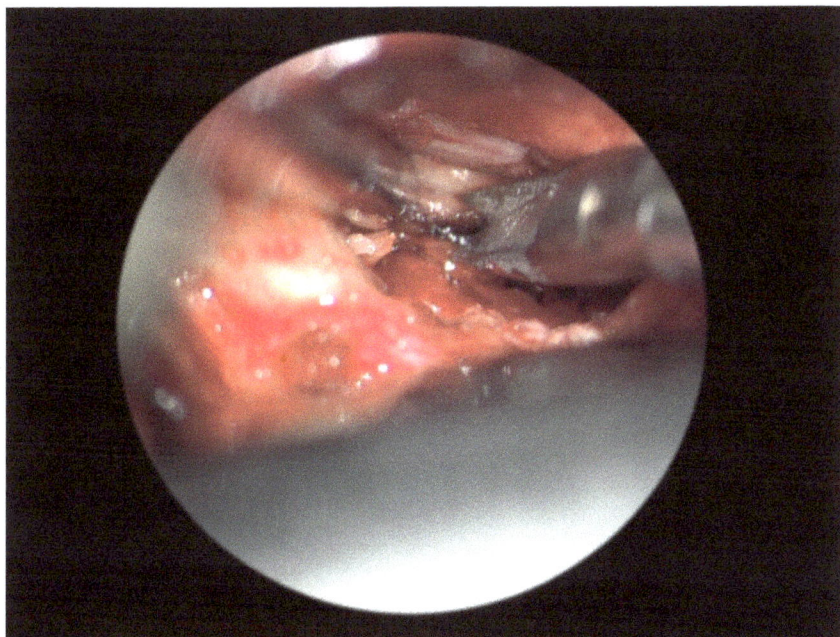

Fig. 3.35: Cut the coagulated vessels with sharp microscissors

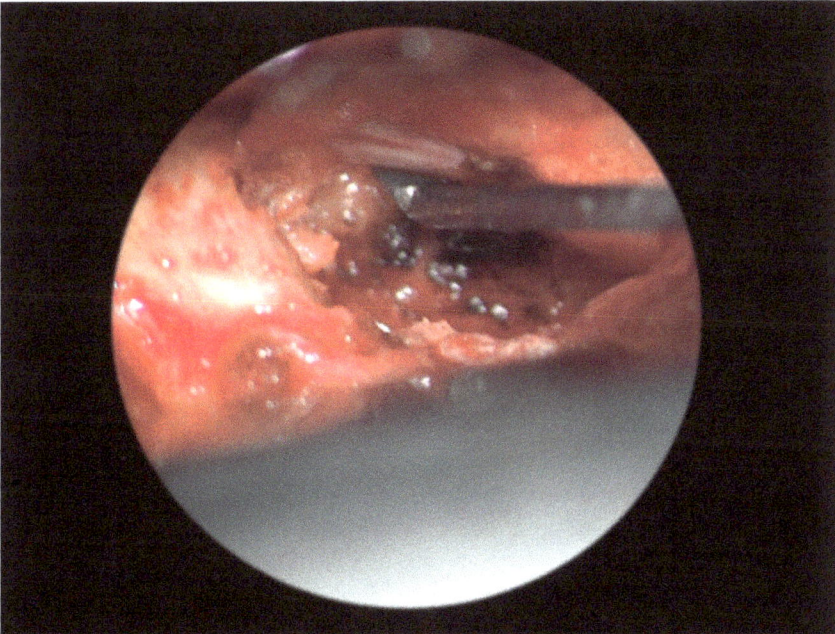

Fig. 3.36: Retract the stretched nerve root with a small dissector or rasparator. This step helps in understanding the extent of the stretch of the nerve root by the underlying disc prolapse

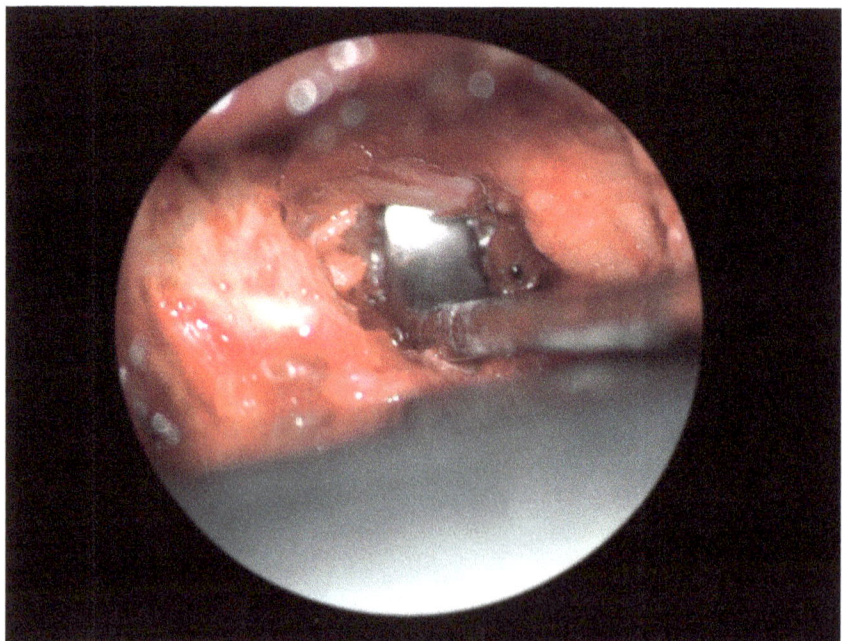

Fig. 3.37: Retract the nerve root with a standard angulated nerve root retractor towards midline gently

Step 5-Exposure of disc space: The nerve root should be retracted initially with a rasperator and then with a specialized retractor which can also be used to push the annulus down **(Figs 3.38 and 3.39)**. Epidural space is cleared further to expose bulging annulus and disc material. Epidural bleeders are cauterized at this point so that discectomy is done easily. The assistant is advised to keep the nerve root retracted medially with gentle force. The aim is to expose adequate space for easy discectomy **(Fig. 3.40)**.

Step 6-Discectomy and nerve root decompression: Using a number 11 knife annulus is cut in craniocaudal direction **(Fig. 3.41)**. The degenerated disc material protrudes out under pressure and by pressing the annulus down by the retractor more disc material gets extruded **(Figs 3.42 and 3.43)**. Small blunt hooks and sharp hooks are used to deliver these loose degenerated disc fragments under annulus and posterior longitudinal ligament **(Fig. 3.44 to 3.46)**. Disc materials are then removed with disc punches of different sizes **(Figs 3.47 and 3.48)**. The nerve root retractor is adjusted in order to visualize hidden extruded disc material in epidural space. During these maneuvers never retract the nerve superiorly. Sometimes annulotomy can be extended to reduce the bulge and achieve more space to visualize intradiscal region **(Figs 3.49 to 3.51)**. By this time, we can appreciate the lax nerve root.

Operative Techniques with Case Examples | 37

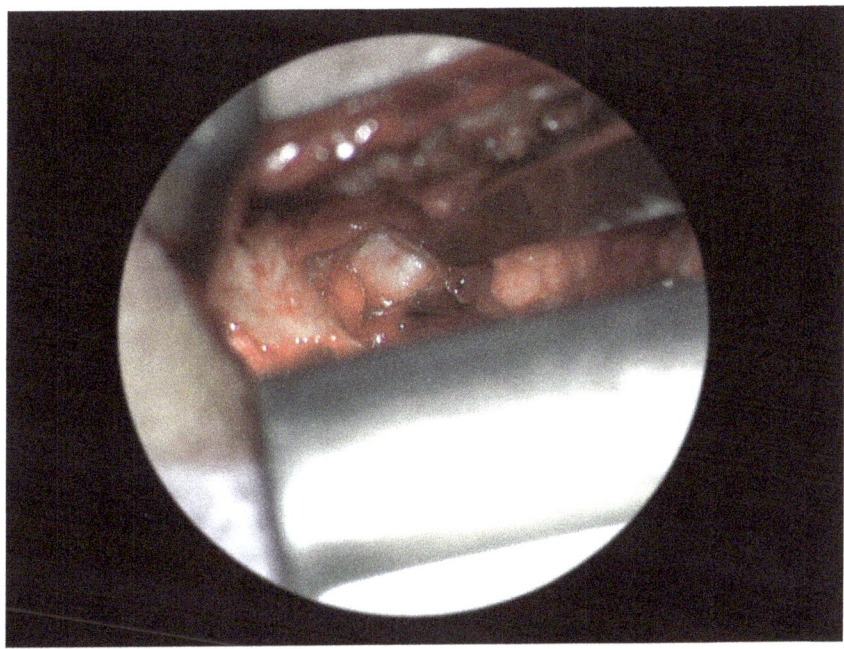

Fig. 3.38: Bulging annulus is well visualized

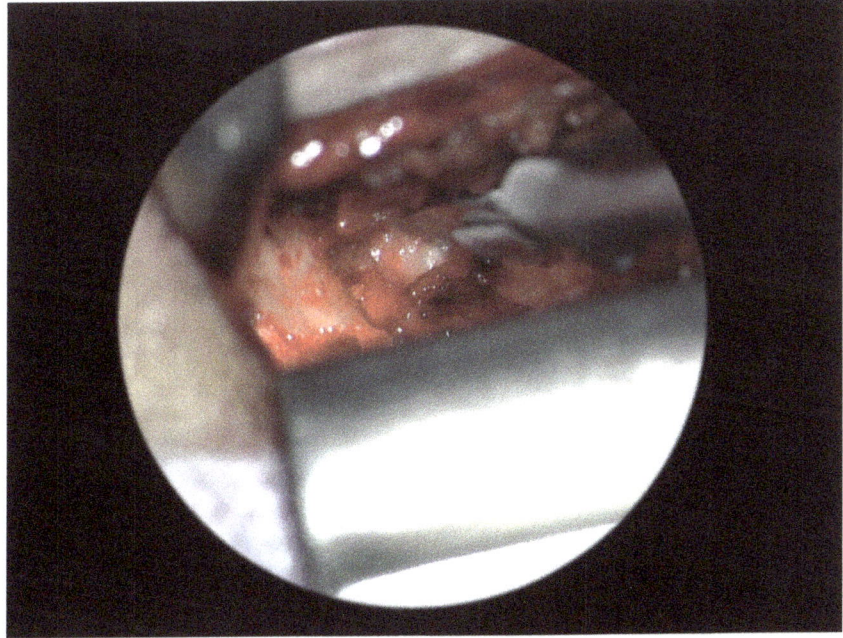

Fig. 3.39: Incise the annulus with No. 11 blade knife craniocaudally

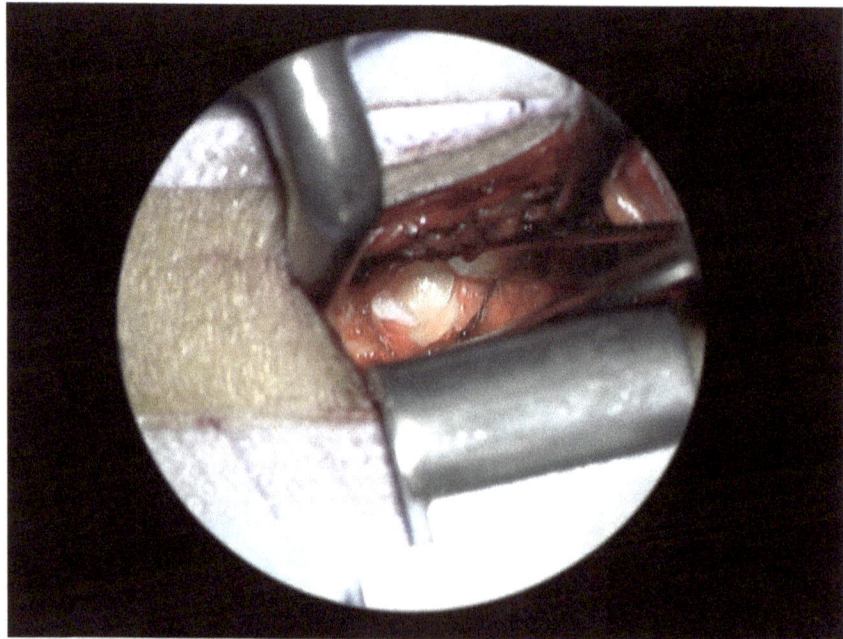

Fig. 3.40: Prolapsed disc material usually comes out under pressure

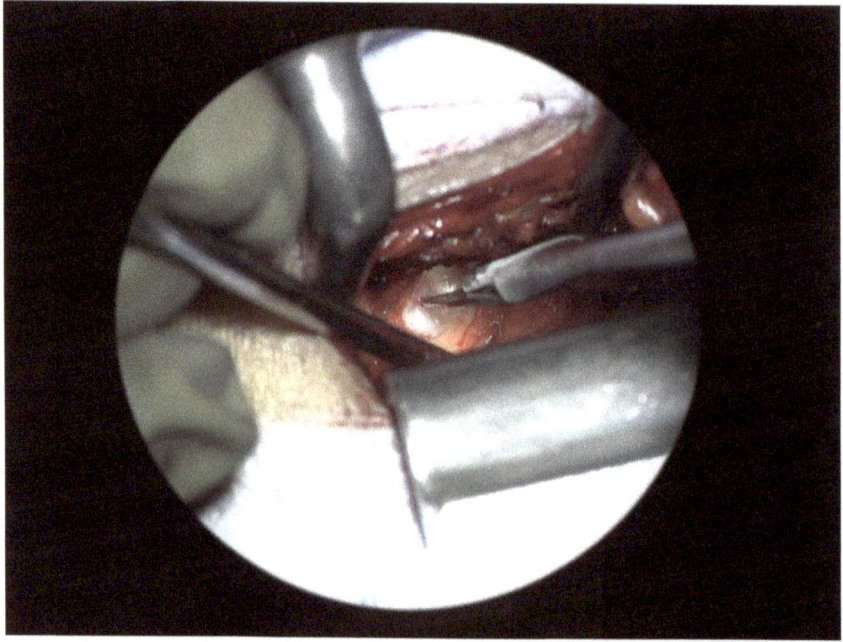

Fig. 3.41: Incision is further extended down

Operative Techniques with Case Examples | 39

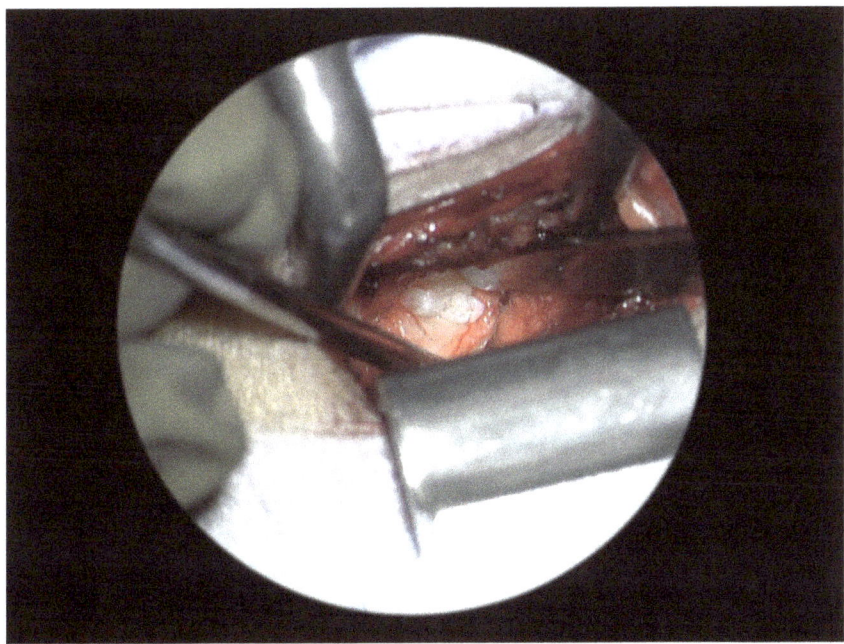

Fig. 3.42: More degenerated disc material pops out

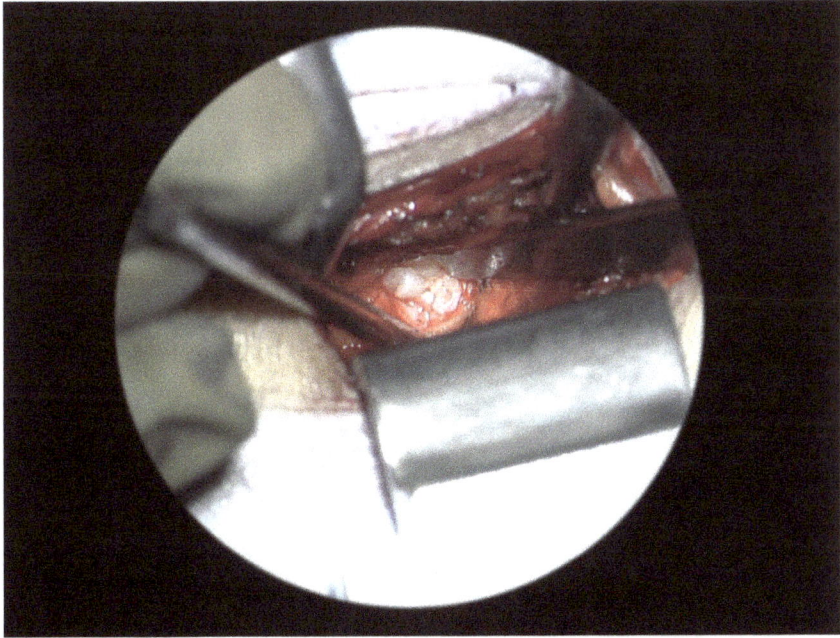

Fig. 3.43: By pushing the annulus with retractor base on the medial side, further disc material could be brought out

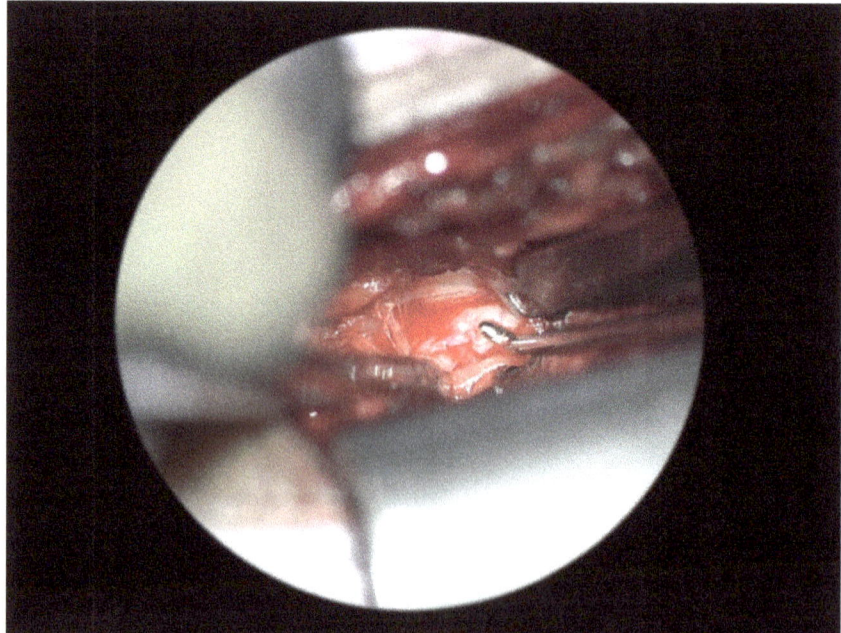

Fig. 3.44: Blunt hook

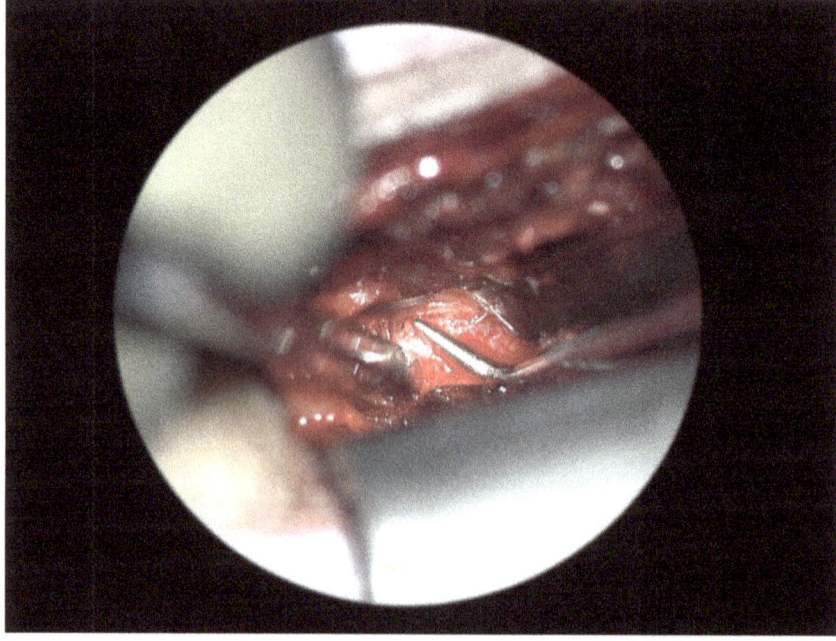

Fig. 3.45: Sharp hooks can now be used to extract the degenerated disc material from under the annulus

Operative Techniques with Case Examples | 41

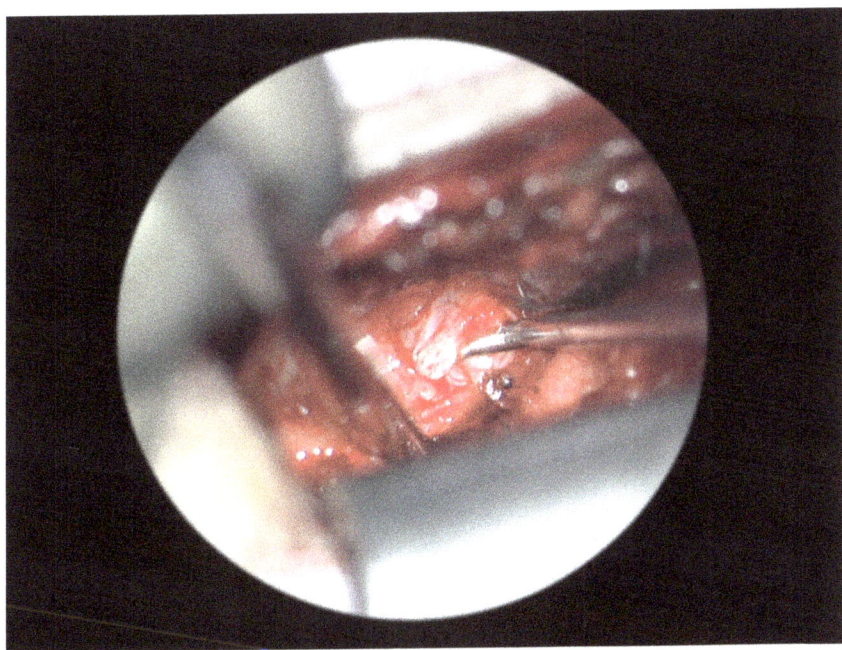

Fig. 3.46: Disc material hooked and pulled out

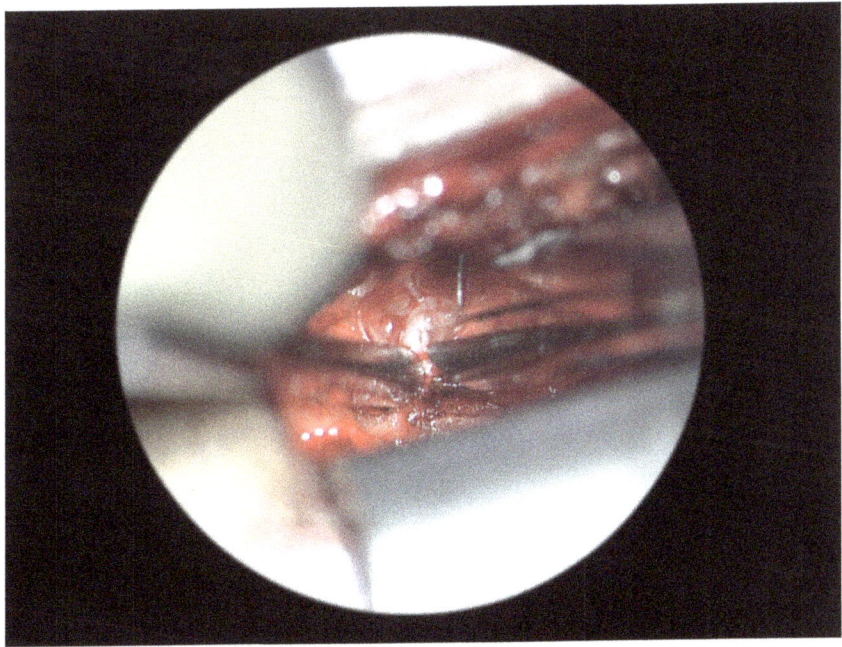

Fig. 3.47: Straight narrow jaws with serration disc punch is used to remove the disc material

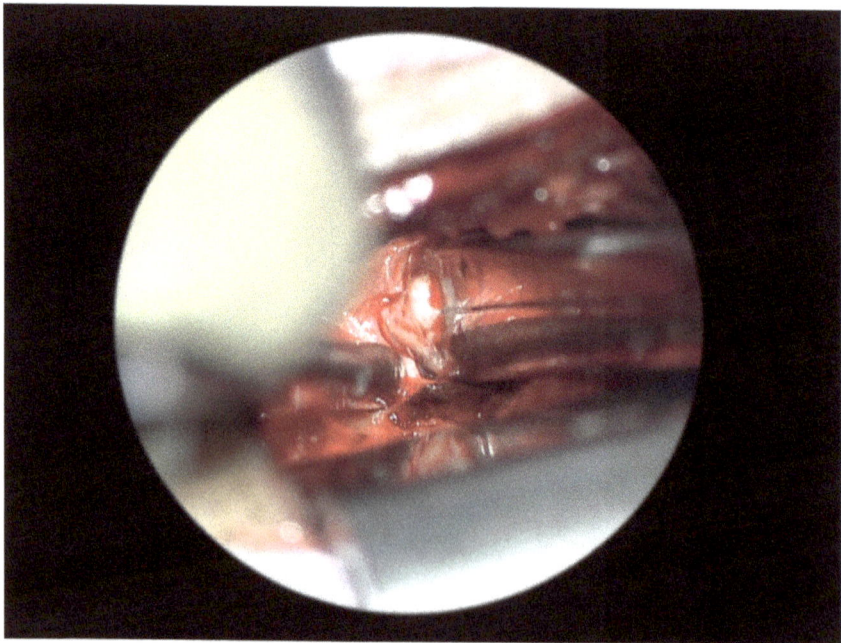

Fig. 3.48: Straight punch is then gently entered in the disc space to remove the intradiscal portion of the free disc material

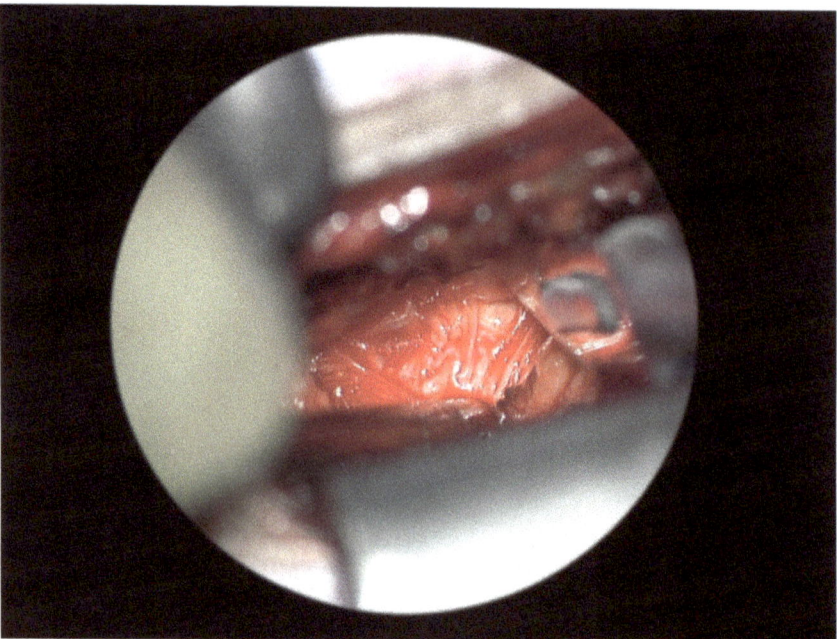

Fig. 3.49: Intradiscal decompression further relaxes the nerve root. Bulging annulus, if present, medially can now be cut to facilitate further removal of free disc material

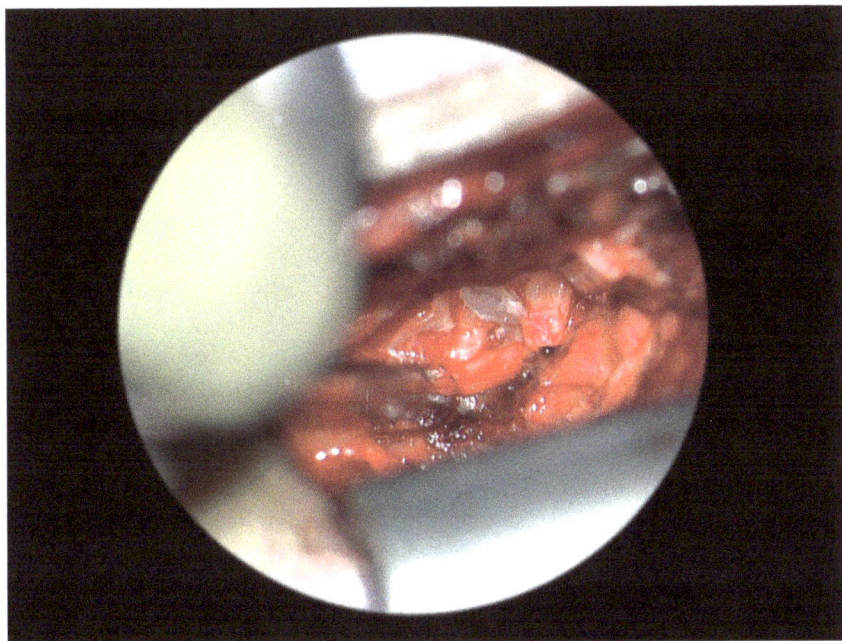

Fig. 3.50: Thorough check should be done to visualize unseen disc material above and below the posterior longitudinal ligament

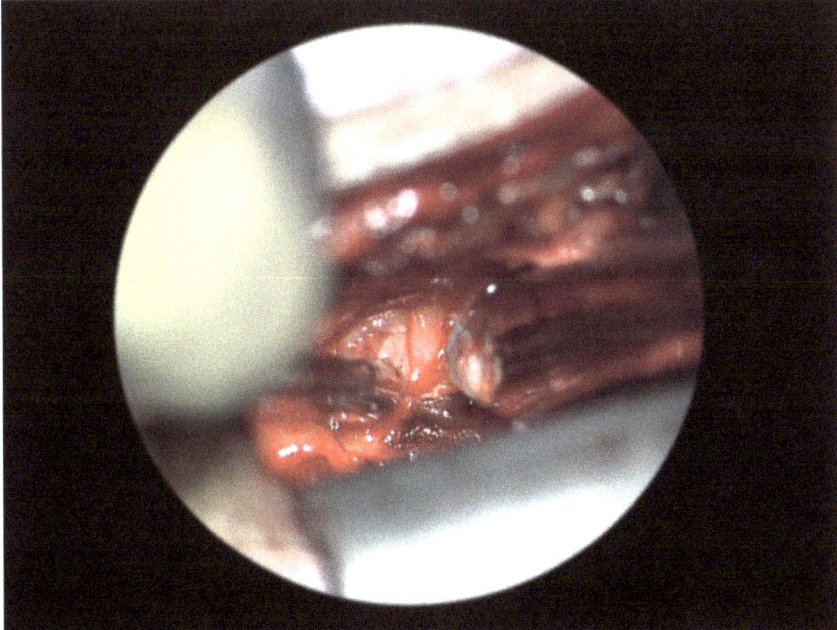

Fig. 3.51: Patiently remove the free disc fragments

Now we can shift the focus in searching free fragments intradiscal space **(Fig. 3.52A)**. This is a very important step and I like to emphasize a few salient technical points. Never use force while inserting the disc punches inside the disc. The annulus and cartilage are slippery and you may end up in inadvertently breaching ventral annulus and even piercing it thus entering in the retroperitoneal region causing damage to major vessels **(Figs 3.52B and 3.52C)**. Many such cases are not reported but heard once in a while. Hence the surgeon should have full control of the disc punch while fishing out free disc fragments in the intradiscal space. Meticulous search must be made in all directions to' fish out 'free fragments **(Figs 3.53 and 3.54)**. Normal tissues should be left alone and no effort should be made to pull them out.

While forward (up) angled punches are used to clear superior region, backward (down) angled punches are used to clear inferior regions of intra-discal space. In conclusion, the 'fish out' technique should be gentle without force but should be complete. This certainly reduces the chance of early recurrent disc prolapse.

A lax nerve root will be seen moving in the canal with respiration and confirm satisfactory decompression **(Figs 3.55 and 3.56)**. A root canal probe can be used to check free nerve in the canal.

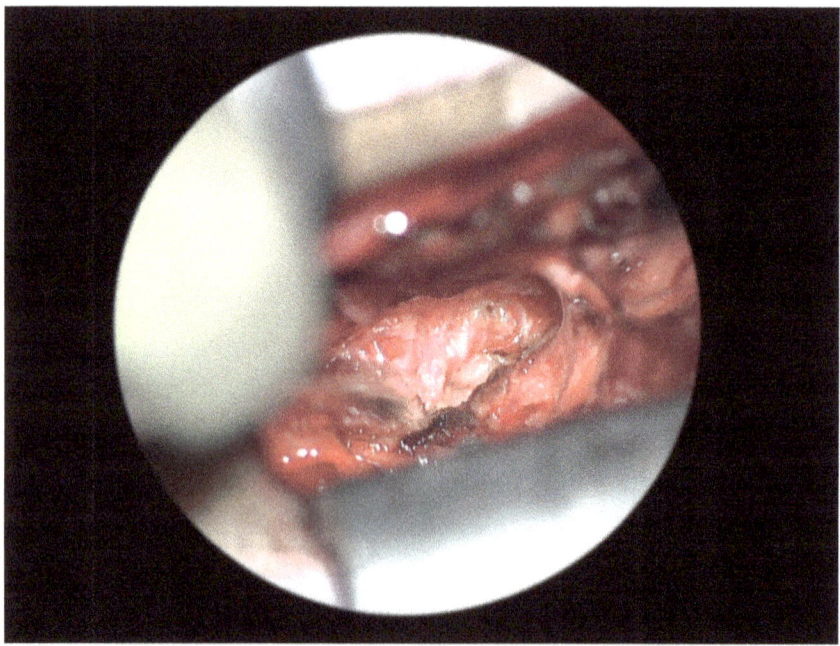

Fig. 3.52A: Surprisingly sometimes more fragments will be seen

Operative Techniques with Case Examples | 45

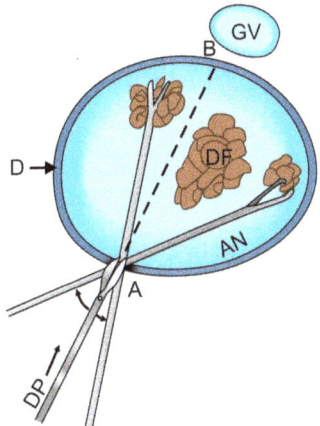

Fig. 3.52B Intra discal 'fishout' (B→ distal annulus)
Abbreviations: A, annulotomy site; AN, annulus; D, disc; DF, degenerated disc fragments; DP, disc punch; GV, great vessels in abdominal cavity

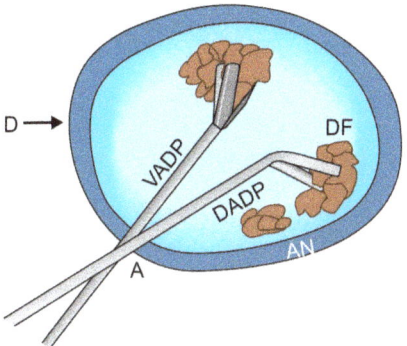

Fig. 3.52C Intra discal 'fishout'
Abbreviations: A, annulotomy site; AN, annulus; D, disc; DF, degenerated disc fragments; DADP, down angled disc punch; UADP, upward angled disc punch

Step 7–Hemostasis and denervation of annulus: Occasionally after discectomy, sometimes, one can encounter batson's plexus bleeding **(Figs 3.57 and 3.58)**. The bleeders should be cauterized. The annulus can be cauterised with low current using microbipolar (This is not mandatory). This actually does thermal denervation of the annulus. A good warm saline wash is given and fat lobules nearby can be pulled to cover the lax nerve root **(Fig. 3.59)**.

Step 8–Closure: Double hook retractor blades are removed and any bleeding from muscle is arrested **(Figs 3.60 and 3.61)**. Usually I keep a small drain over the lamina and bring the tube through a separate stab wound far away. The dorsolumbar fascia is then approximated with number 2-0 vicryl. Subcutaneous layer is approximated with number 2-0 vicryl and a

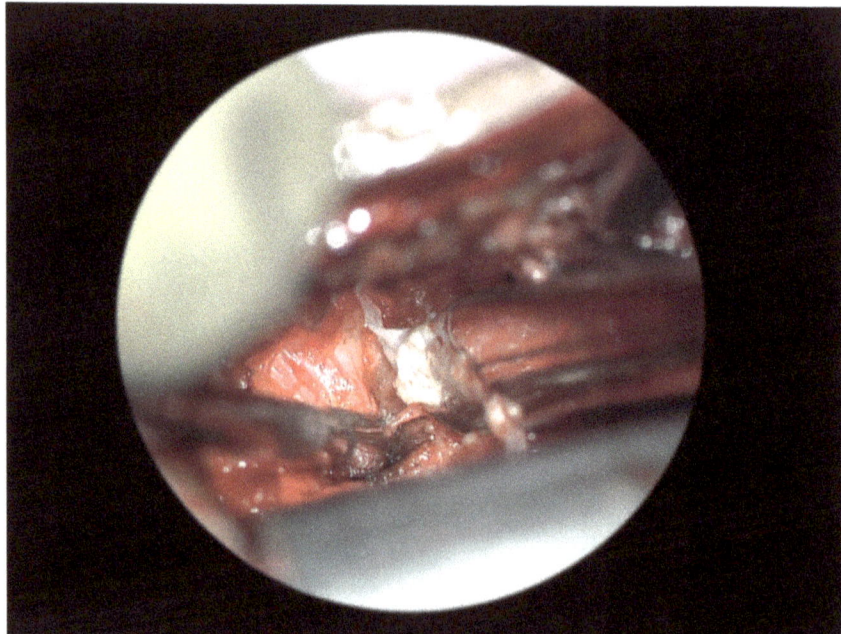

Fig. 3.53: They are meticulously removed

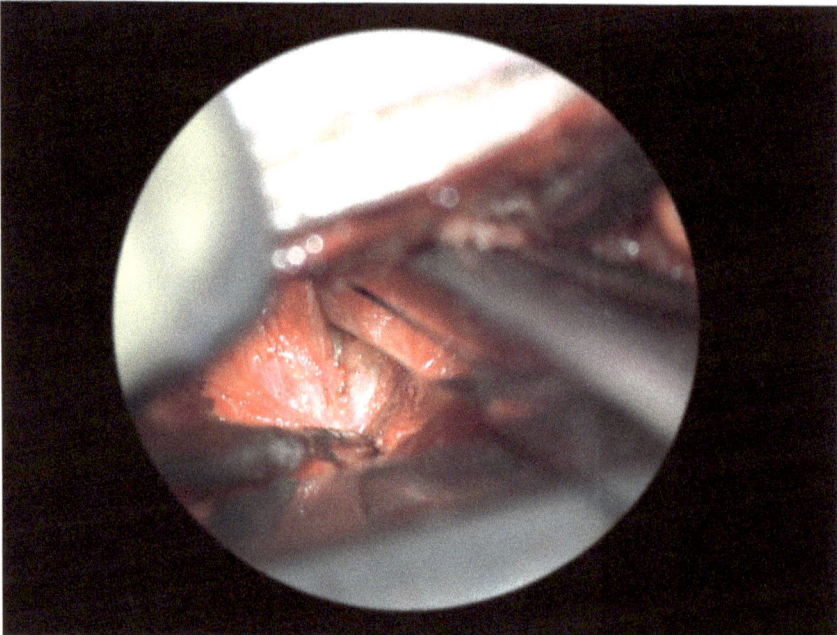

Fig. 3.54: Disc punch is then introduced towards the opposite side gently to 'fish out' deep-seated free fragments. NEVER force be exerted in this step. The proprioceptive sense of the surgeon's hand is vital here

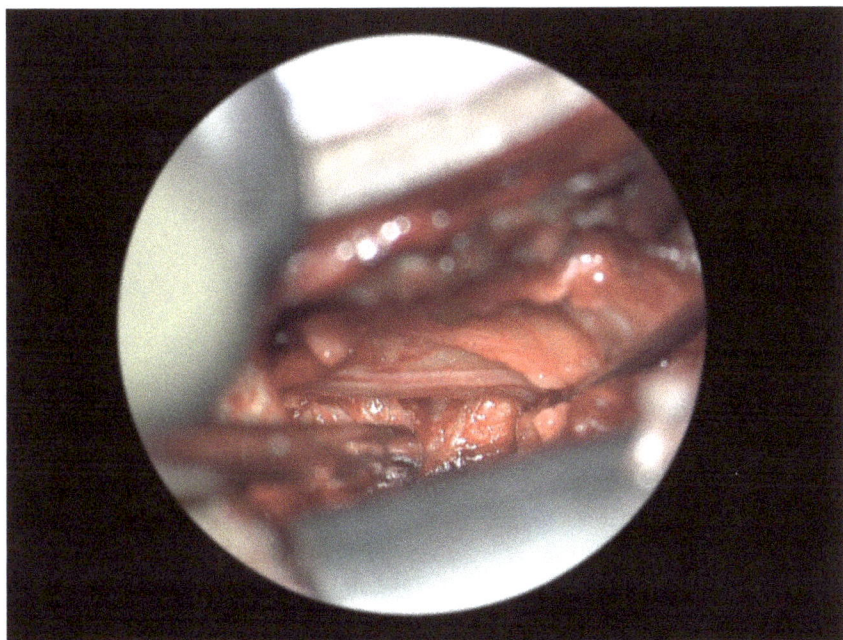

Fig. 3.55: After removing the disc material, the nerve root retractor is released. The lax nerve root is seen to full length

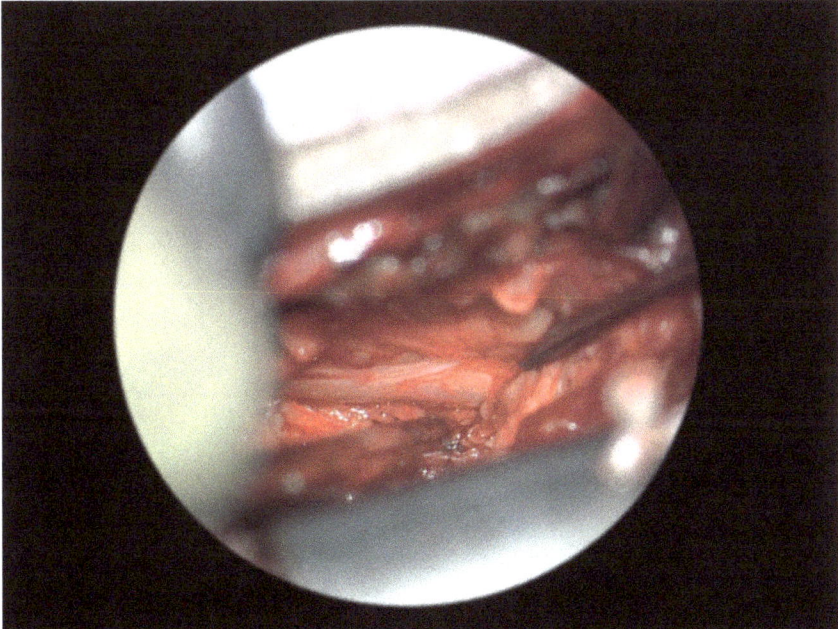

Fig. 3.56: Nerve root is examined under higher magnification. Good movement of the root is appreciated. This indicates satisfactory and adequate decompression

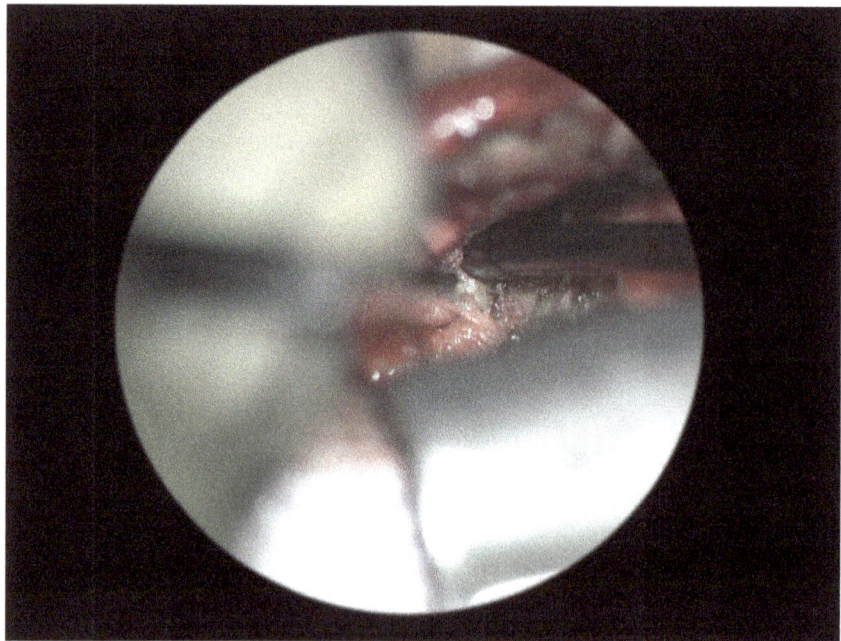

Fig. 3.57: The annular edges can be coagulated with micro tip bipolar with low current. This denerve the annulus

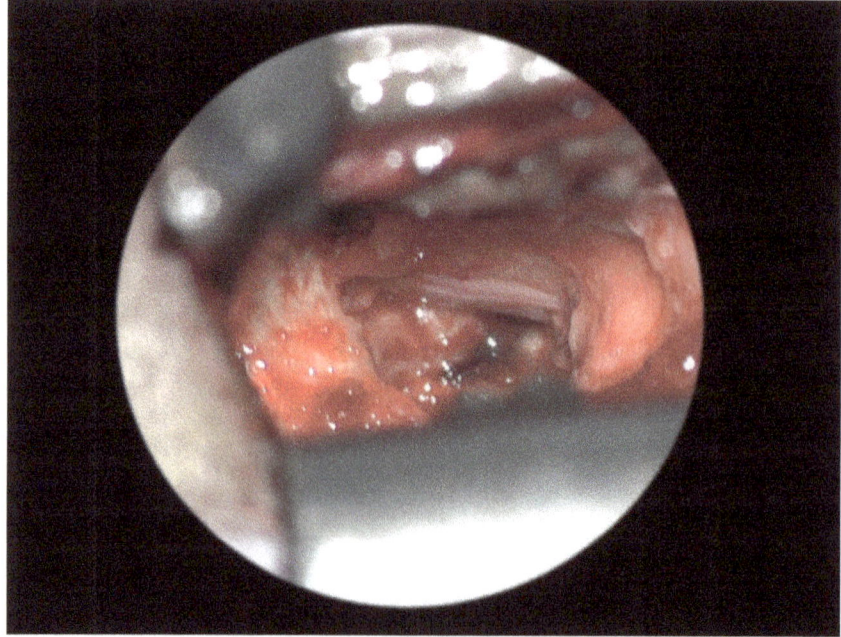

Fig. 3.58: Saline wash is given

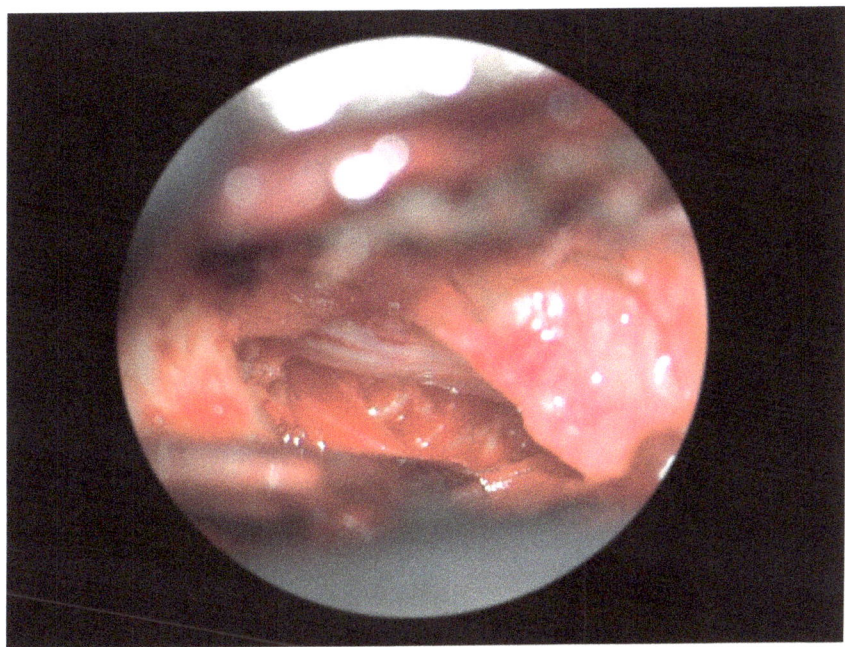

Fig. 3.59: Fat lobules mobilized over the nerve root

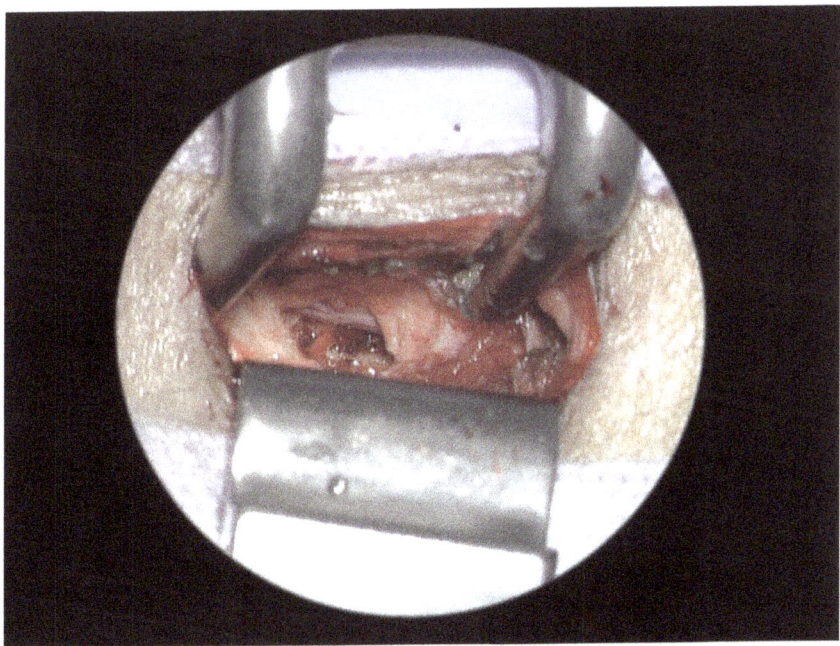

Fig. 3.60: Entire wound is inspected again before closure

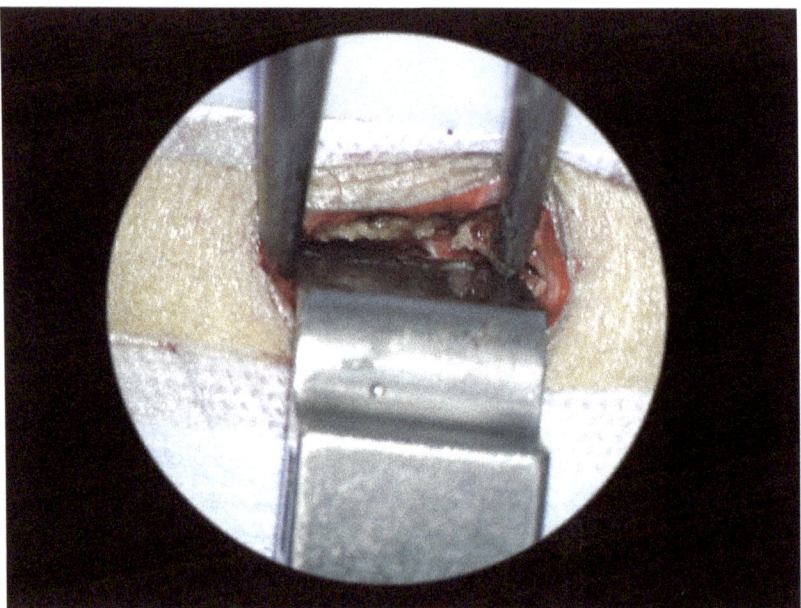

Fig. 3.61: Double-hook retractor is removed

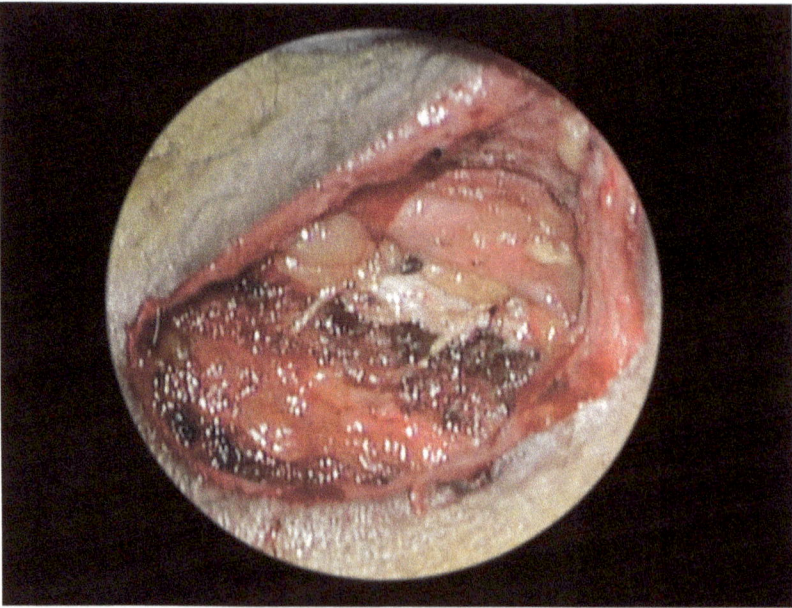

Fig. 3.62: Dorsolumbar fascia approximated with Vicryl No. 2 after placing a drain below the muscle over the lamina

subcuticular 3-0 Monocryl suture is done to approximate the skin incision **(Figs 3.62 to 3.64)**. A small elastoplaster is then applied over the wound. (In terms of usage of epidural steroids, local anesthetic agents and antibiotics, refer to chapter 6).

Operative Techniques with Case Examples | 51

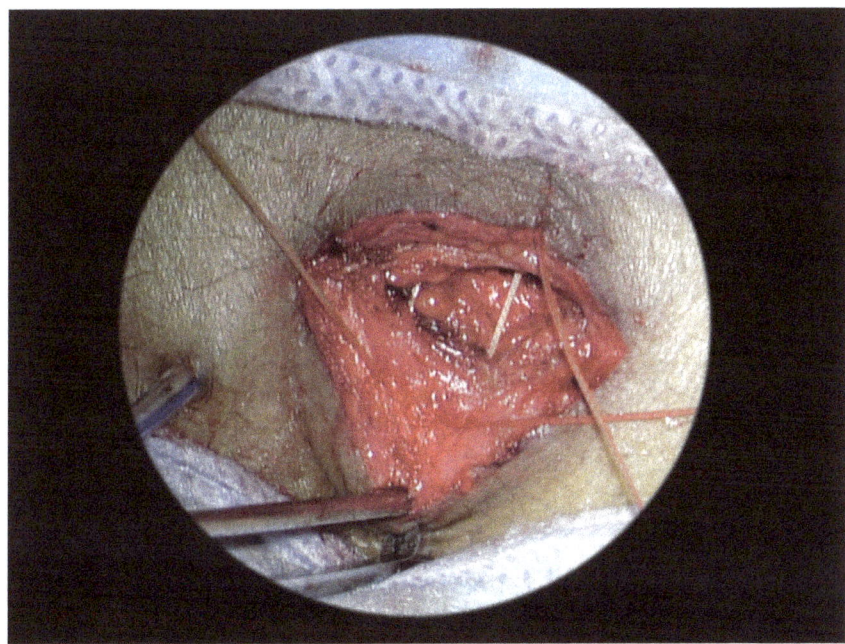

Fig. 3.63: Subcutaneous approximation done with No. 2 Vicryl

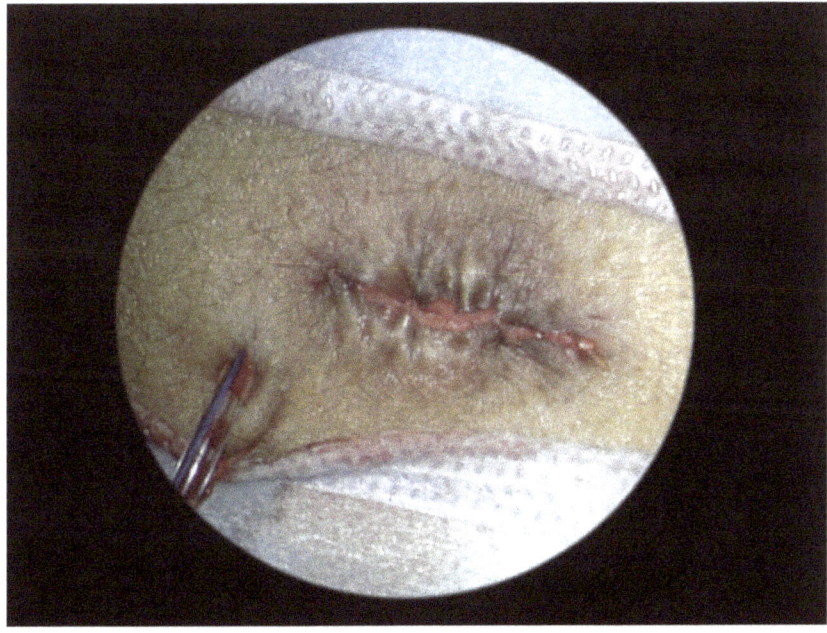

Fig. 3.64: Subcuticular approximation done with monofilament. Drain tube fixed to the shin

Centrolateral Large Disc Prolapse with Lateral Canal Stenosis

Case example: A large wide central and lateral disc prolapse with lateral canal stenosis on right side with thickened ligamentum flavum.

Clinical status: Severe sciatica right leg and back pain **(Figs 3.65 and 3.66)**.

Whenever there is a degenerative disc bulge, lateral canal stenosis, thick ligamentum flavum, severe nerve root compression and associated with narrow interlaminar space, then the lateral canal should be decompressed completely by deroofing it along with discectomy.

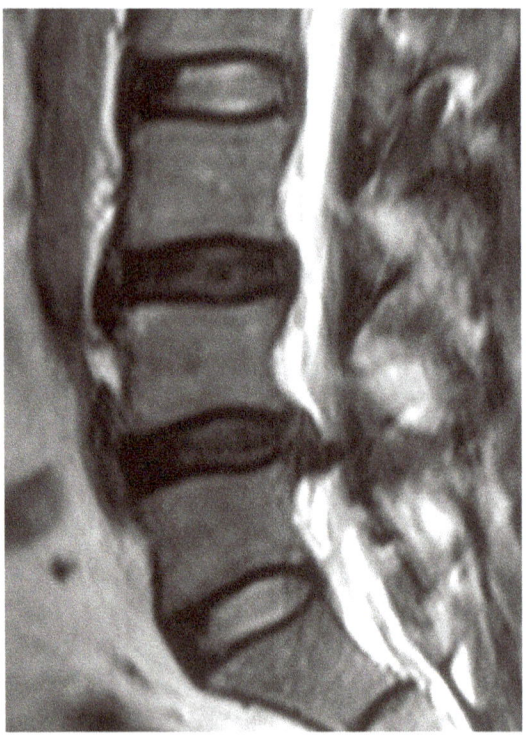

Fig. 3.65: MRI sagittal view showing the large disc prolapse at L_4/L_5 level

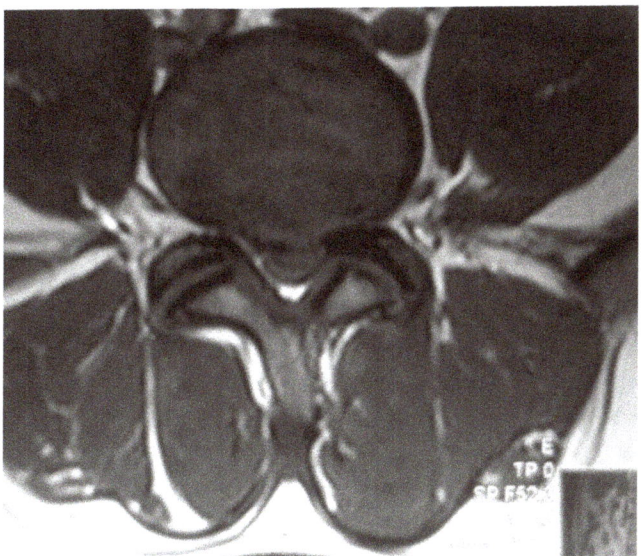

Fig. 3.66: MRI axial view showing a wide and large disc prolapse at central and lateral region with lateral canal stenosis

Operative Procedure (Fig. 3.67A)

Step 1–Exposure of interlaminar space and the bony structures around: The technique is same as explained in earlier case. Surgeon can note the following: Very narrow interlaminar space means all bony structures that border it are crowded **(Figs 3.67B and 3.68)**. All these bony structures are well-dissected and delineated. Soft tissues are removed and the ligamentum flavum is exposed **(Fig. 3.69)**.

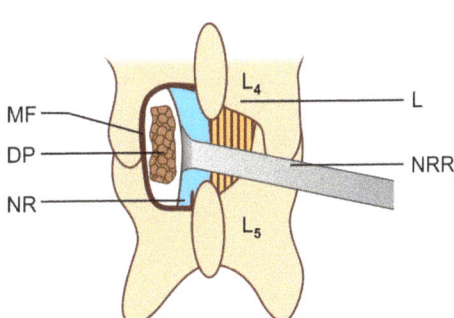

Fig. 3.67A
Abbreviations: DP, disc prolapse; L, lamina; MF, medial facetectomy; NR, nerve root; NRR, nerve root retractor

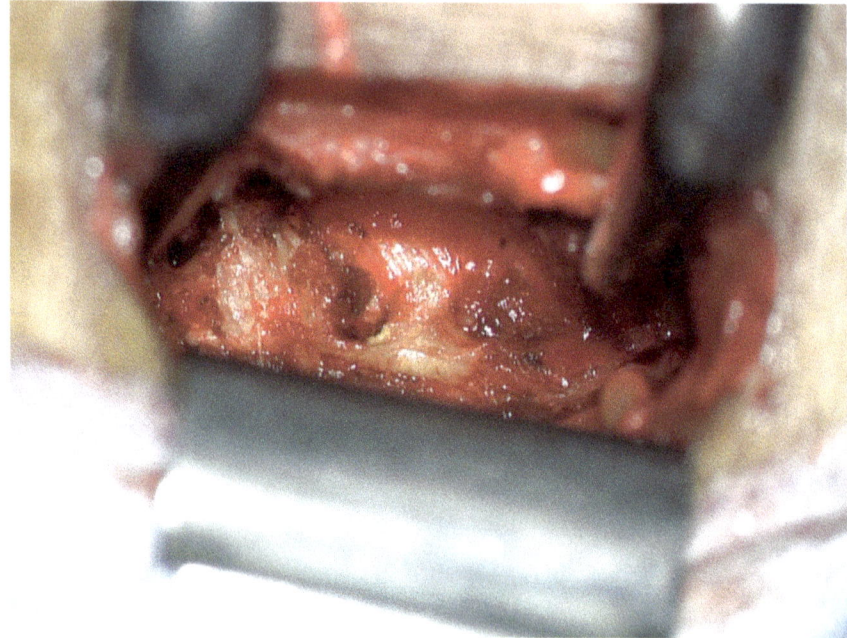

Fig. 3.67B: Soft tissues should be removed well. Interlaminar space exposed

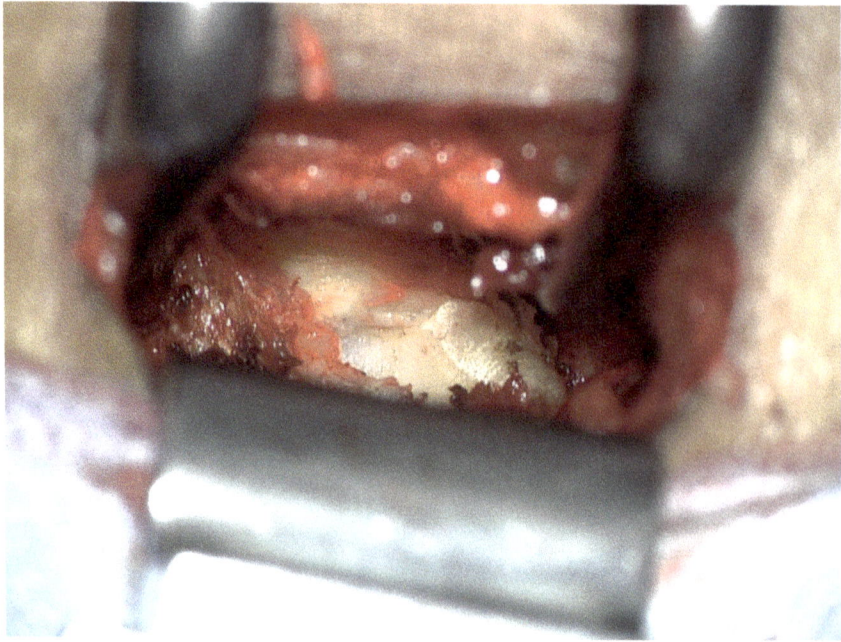

Fig. 3.68: Note the narrow interlaminar space due to crowding of the sloping thick lamina of upper vertebra and superior facet of inferior vertebra

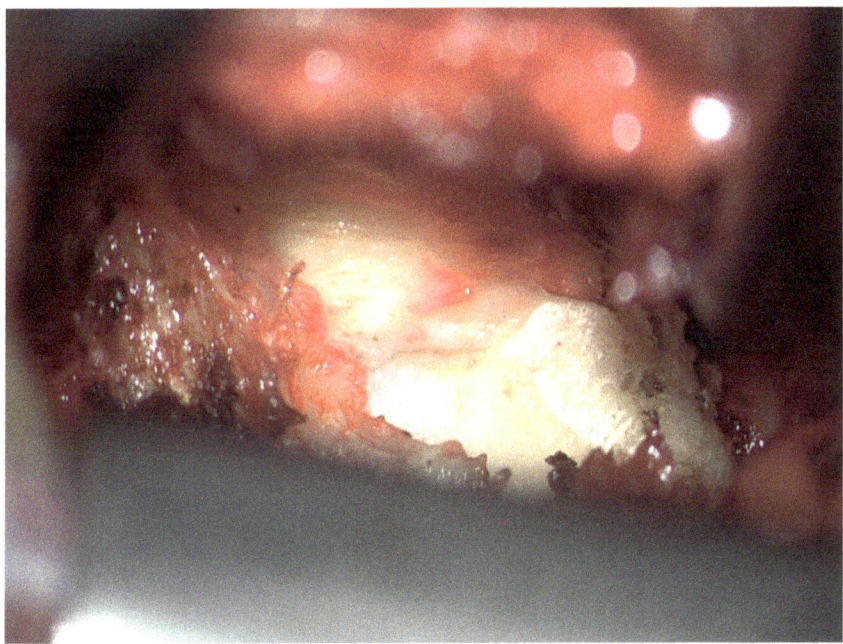

Fig. 3.69: Magnified view also shows the narrow lamina of inferior vertebra

Step 2-Widening of interlaminar space and lateral canal deroofing: Using a high speed drill and diamond burr, the inferior half of upper vertebra **(Fig. 3.70)** and medial 1/3rd of its inferior facet is drilled out first **(Figs 3.71 and 3.72)**. Once the inner table is thinned out, they are removed with number 1 Kerrison punch **(Figs 3.73 to 3.77)**. After the medial 1/3rd of inferior facet is removed, superior facet of lower vertebra will be visualized and the same can be drilled out with ease and then excised now **(Figs 3.78 to 3.80)**. Drilling is further continued over upper half of lower lamina **(Fig. 3.81)**.

Using Kerrison punches from 1 to 3, the thinned out bones are removed **(Fig. 3.82)**. Care should be taken while removing the 1/3rd of superior facet of lower vertebra since the nerve root is usually very close in a compromised state. Ligamentum flavum gets detached in the process of excising the upper laminar border of lower vertebra **(Fig. 3.83)**. The buckled and thick ligamentum flavum is now lifted **(Fig. 3.84)** and removed completely **(Figs 3.85 and 3.86)**.

Step 3-Nerve root decompression: Epidural space is now inspected and nerve root is identified **(Fig. 3.87)**. Fat, Batson's plexus vessels and soft tissues are taken care. The annular bulging and stretched (compressed) nerve root over disc space is delineated **(Figs 3.88 and 3.89)**. The nerve root is retracted medially **(Figs 3.90 and 3.91)** and bulging thick annulus is cut widely in all directions **(Figs 3.92 and 3.93)**.

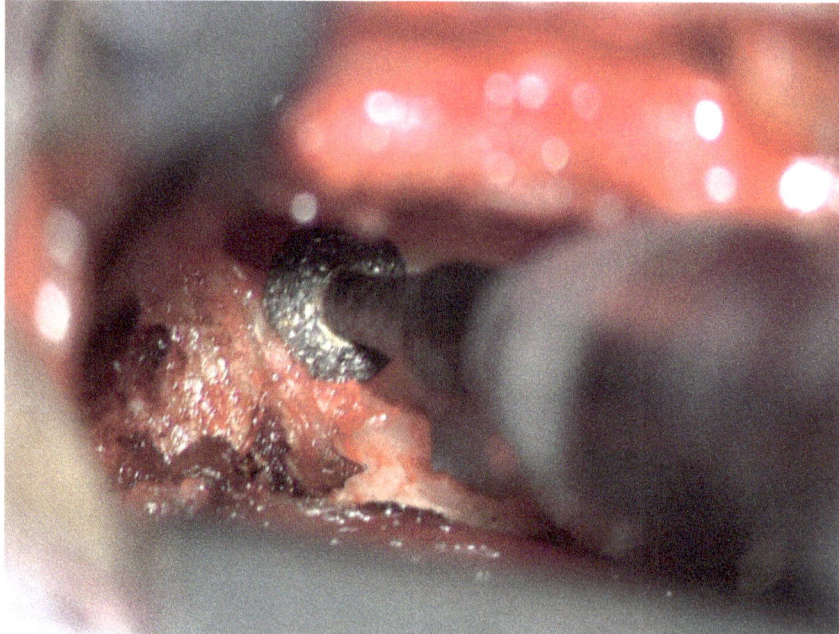

Fig. 3.70: Now, drill the inferior border of upper lamina

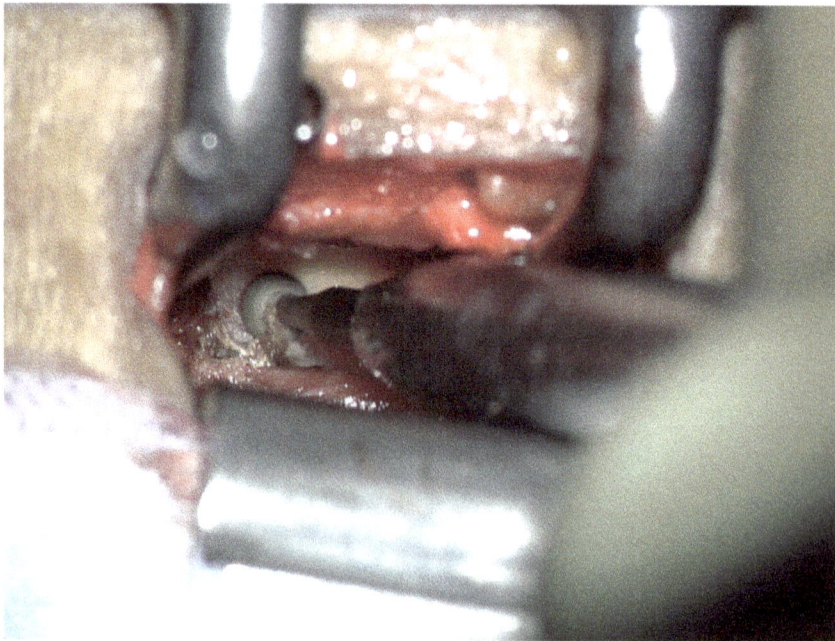

Fig. 3.71: Drill the entire length of the lamina and its junction with the inferior facet of upper vertebra

Operative Techniques with Case Examples | 57

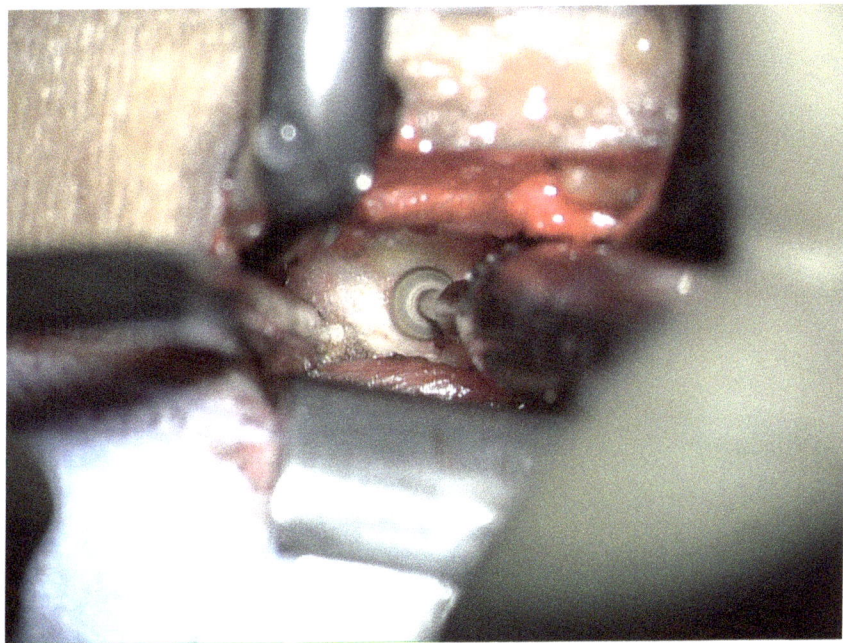

Fig. 3.72: Medial one-third of the inferior facet is drilled out with a diamond burr

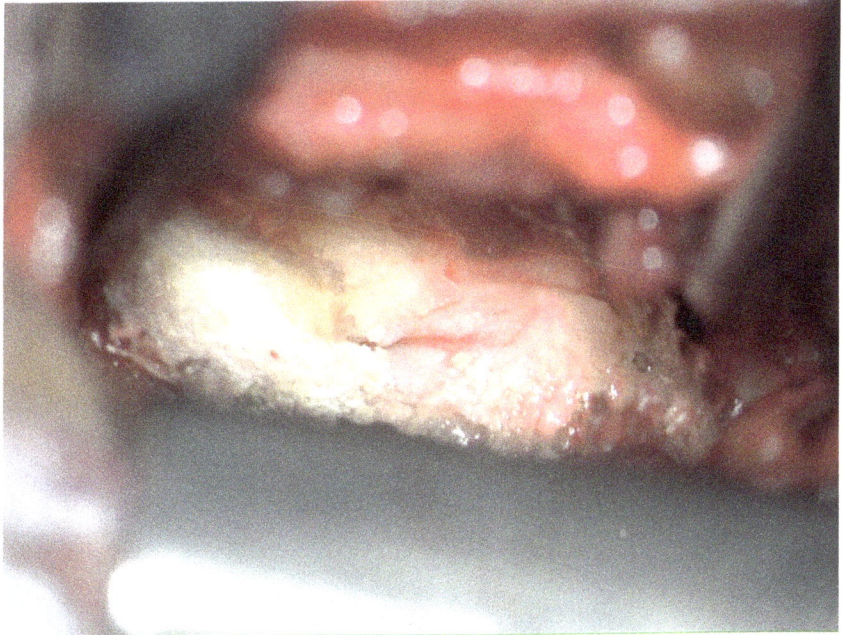

Fig. 3.73: Drilling should be done until the inner table is made thin

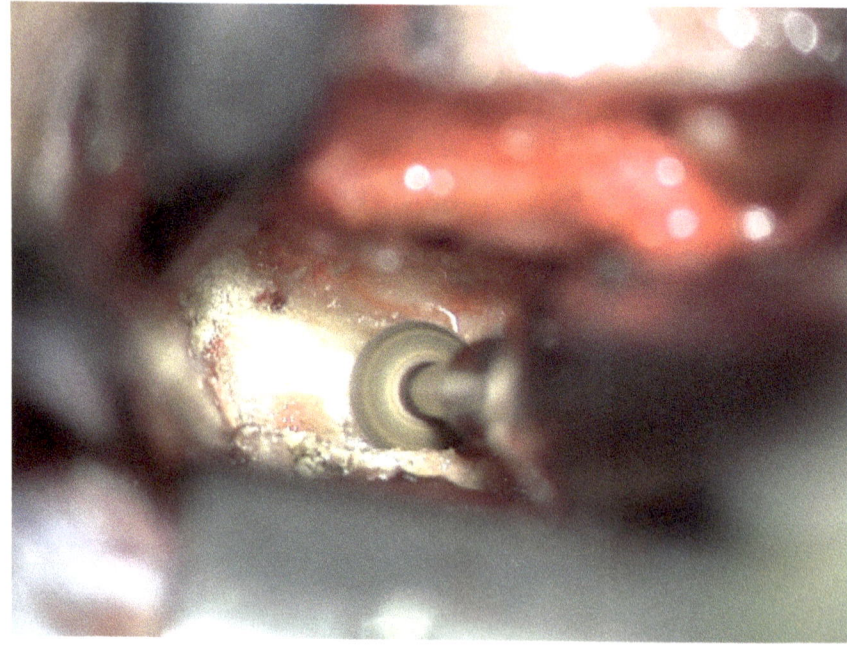

Fig. 3.74: Subsequently, drilling should be continued over the medial one-third of the superior facet of inferior vertebra

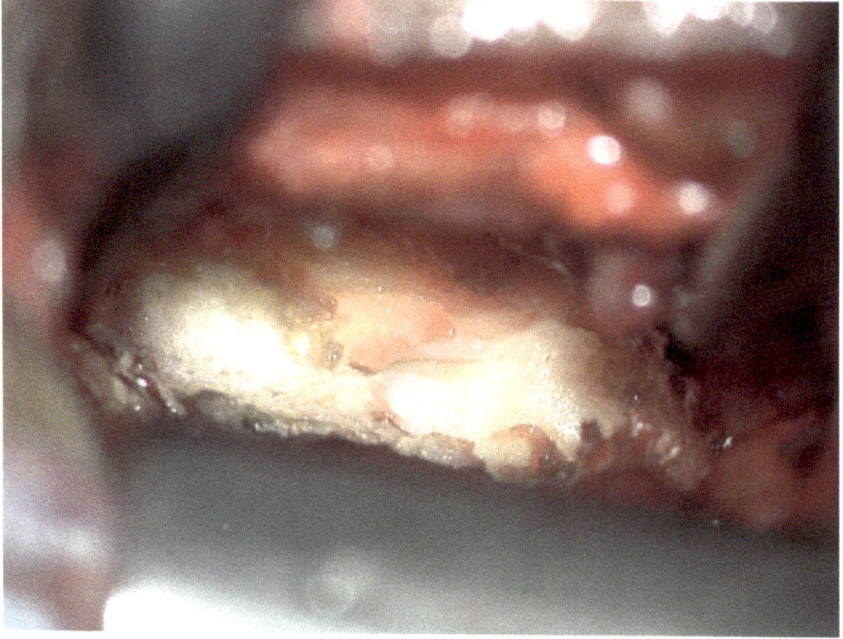

Fig. 3.75: Magnified view of the drilled out facets

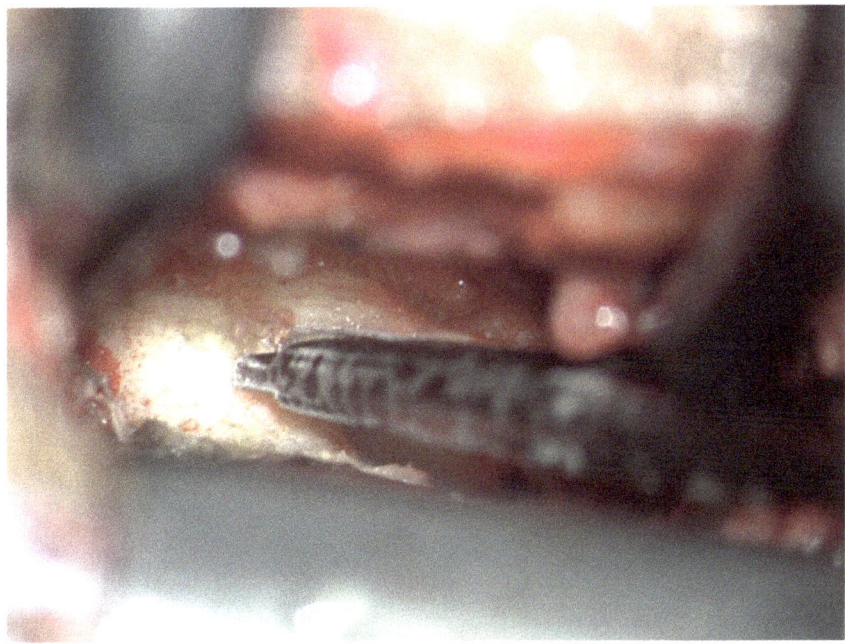

Fig. 3.76: With No.1 Kerrison punch, excise the thin lamina

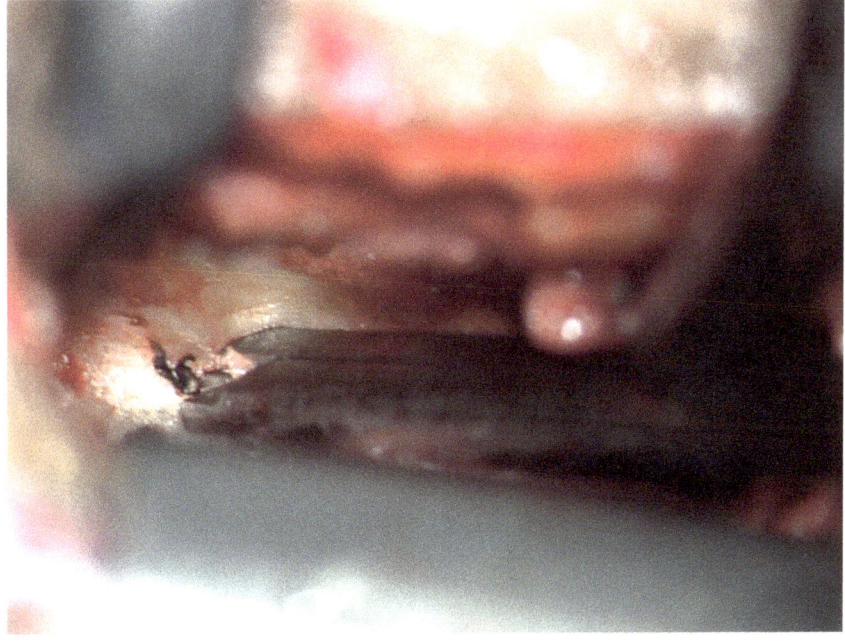

Fig. 3.77: Continue excising the medial one-third of the facet

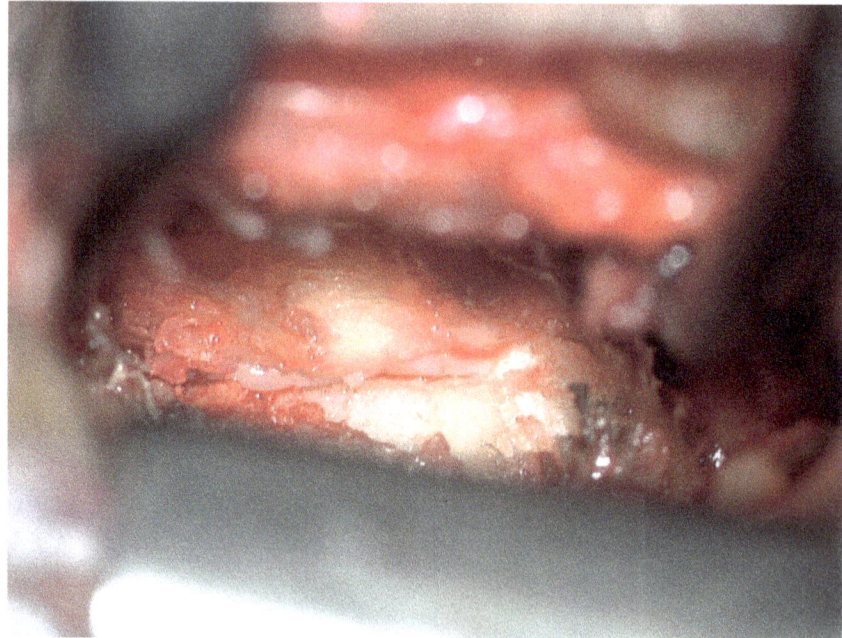

Fig. 3.78: Here underlying thick ligamentum flavum gives a good layer of buffer from the thecal sac (dura). Often they are seen bulging

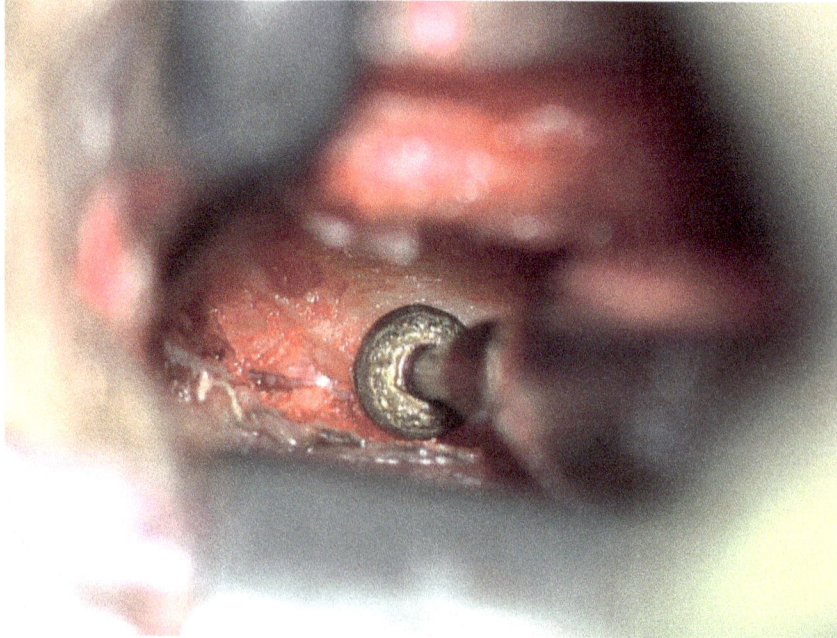

Fig. 3.79: Further drilling is needed to get more widening of the space. This is vital for lateral canal decompression

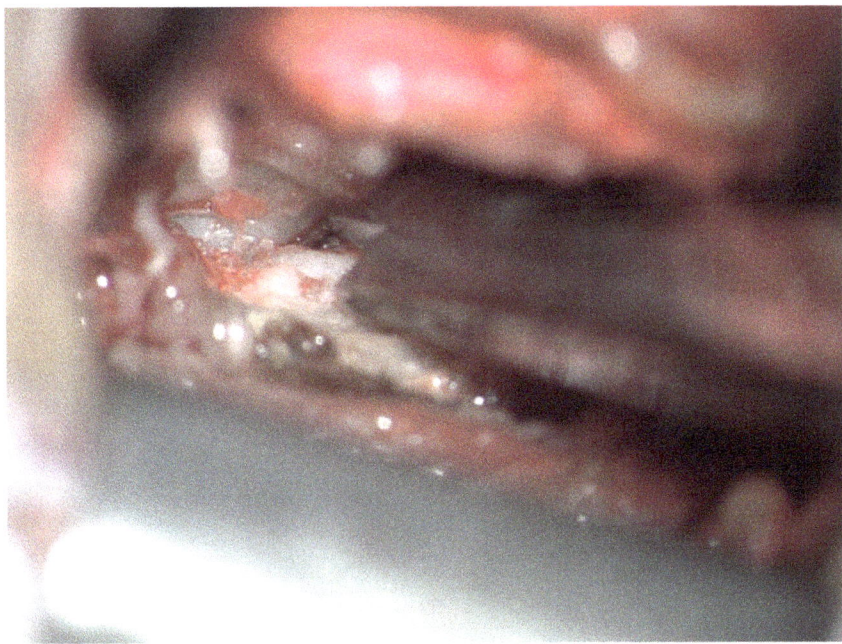

Fig. 3.80: Now, remove the medial one-third of lower facet (superior facet of inferior vertebra)

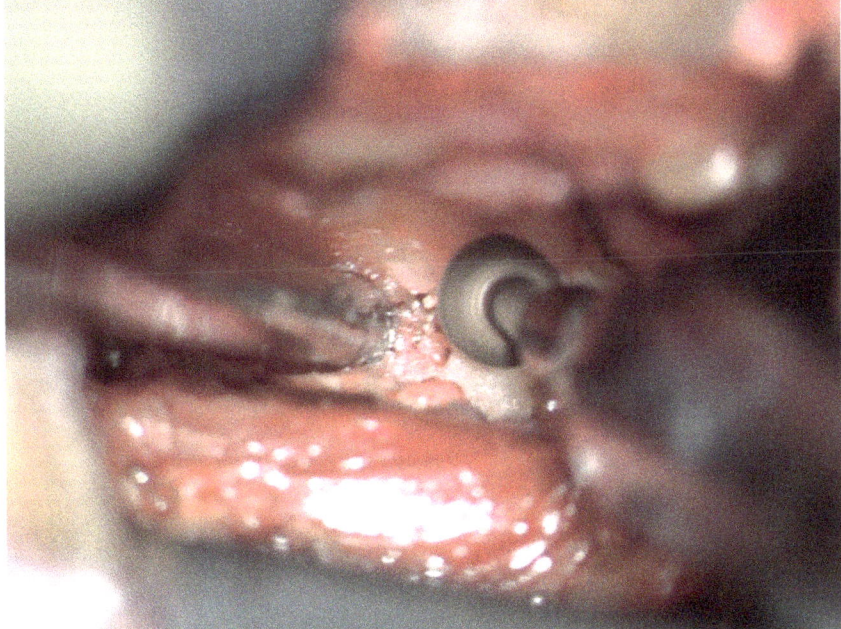

Fig. 3.81: Drill out the superior border of the inferior lamina

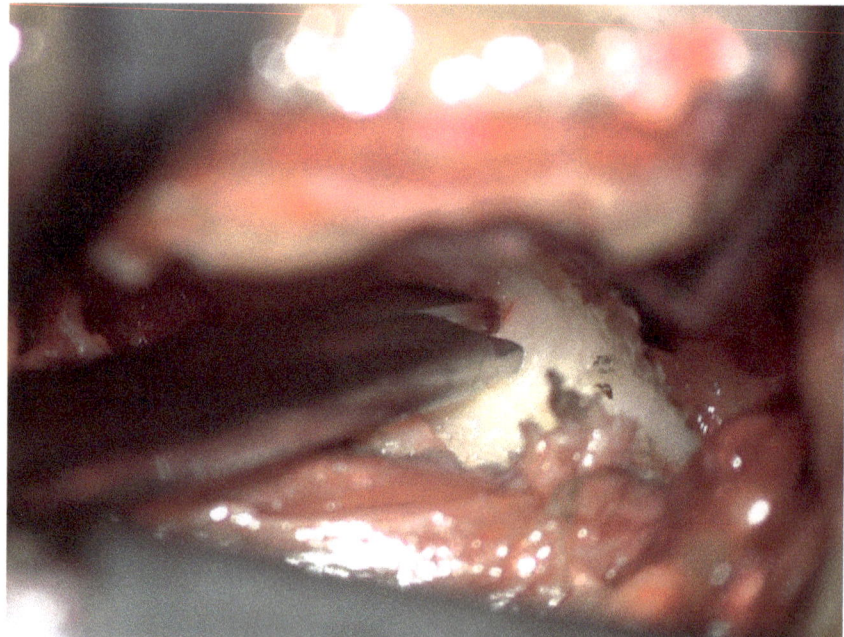

Fig. 3.82: After excising the medial one-third of the lower facet, continue excising the upper one-third of lower lamina

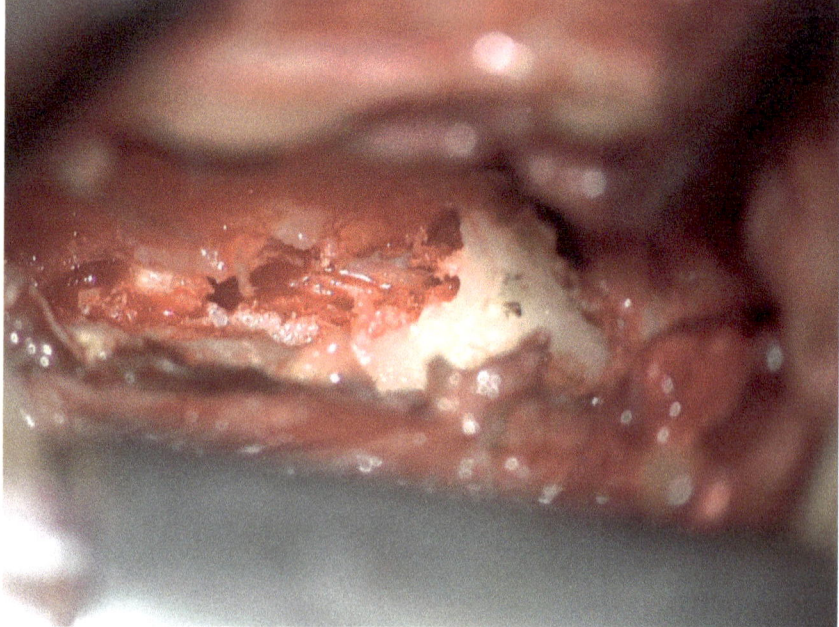

Fig. 3.83: The ligamentum flavum attached to the upper border of lower lamina gets detached automatically thus exposing the extradural space. Here, there is no buffer between bone and dura

Operative Techniques with Case Examples | 63

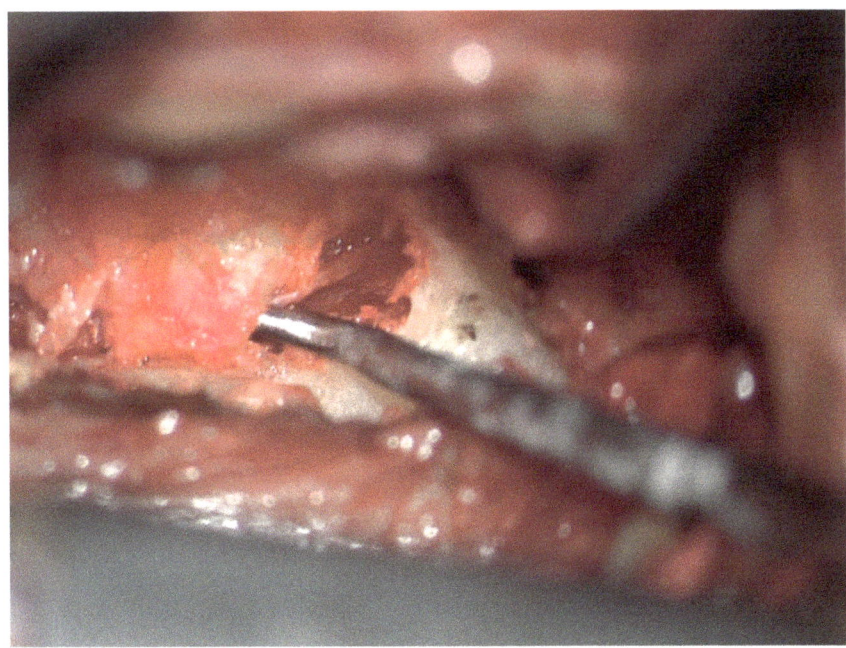

Fig. 3.84: Lift the thickened buckled ligament with a hook

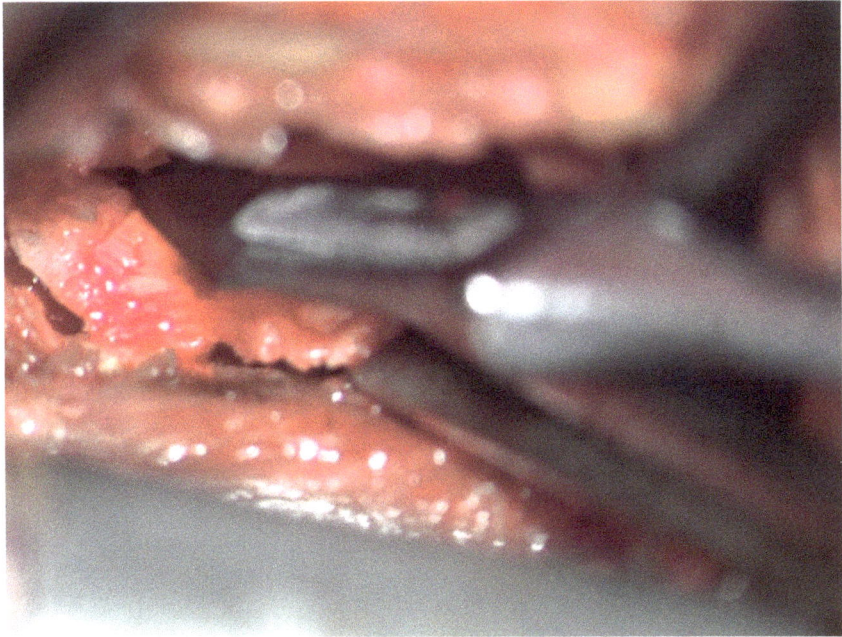

Fig. 3.85: Cut with No. 11 blade while the ligament is lifted from the dura underneath

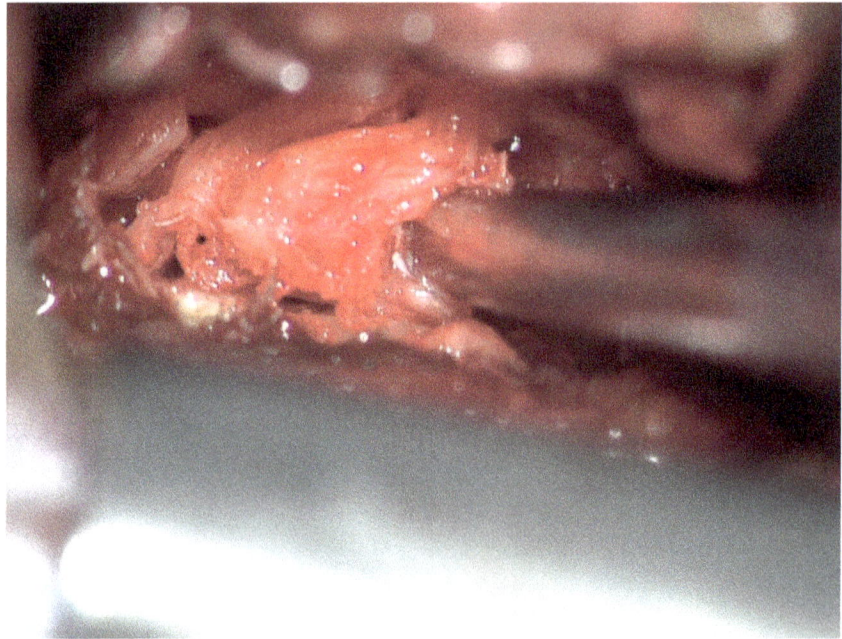

Fig. 3.86: Ligamentum flavum is then excised with Kerrison punches

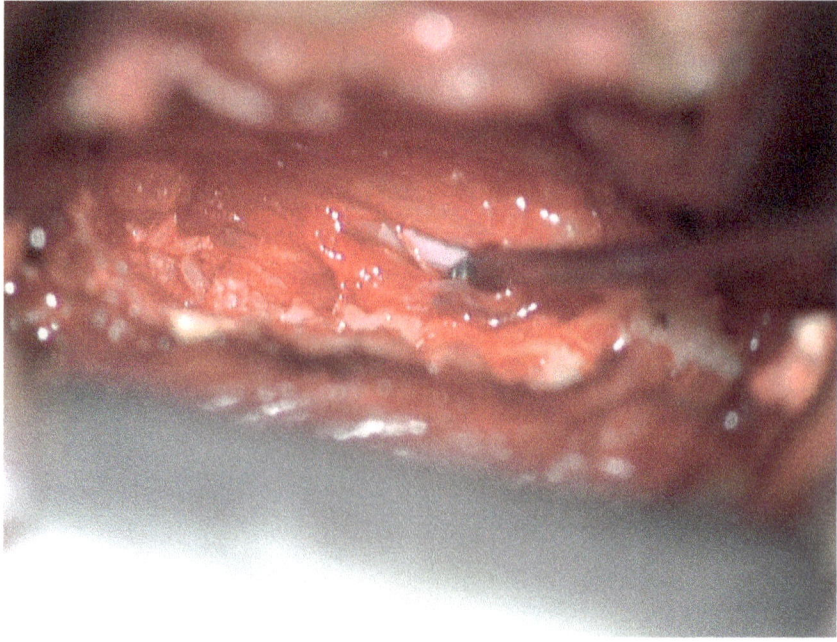

Fig. 3.87: Stretched out nerve root seen along with fat and small vessels in the extradural space

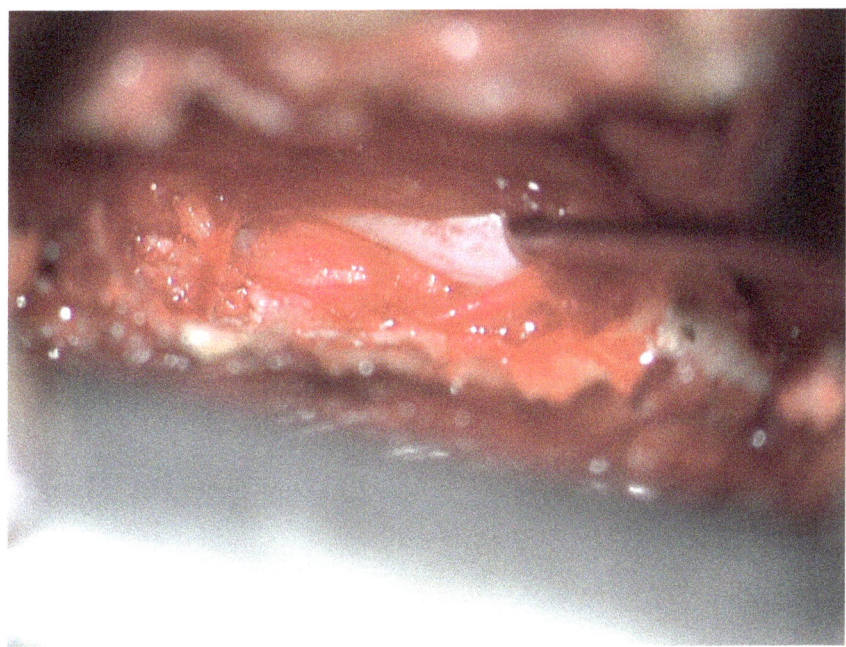

Fig. 3.88: Inspect the nerve root well and assess the disc bulge by its stretch

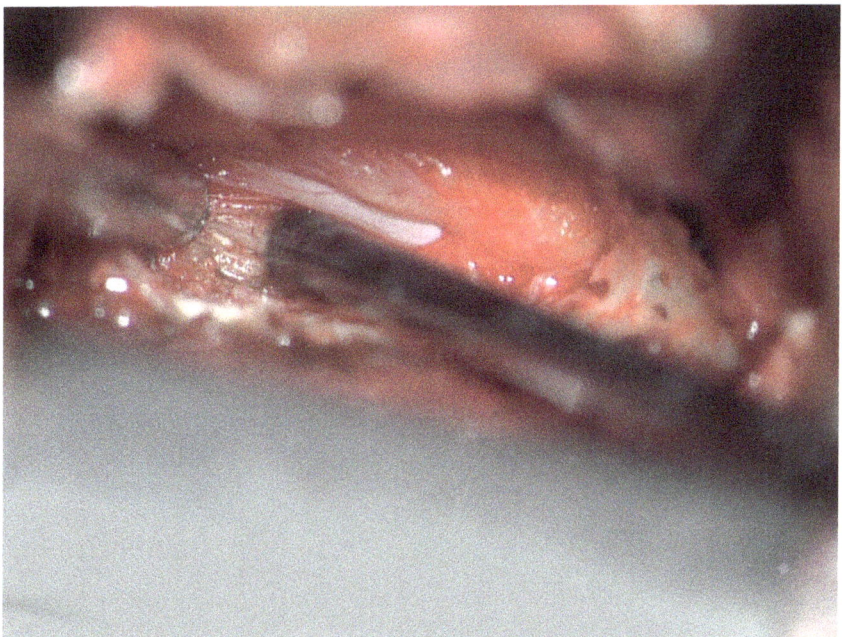

Fig. 3.89: Cauterize the epidural vessels with low current bipolar

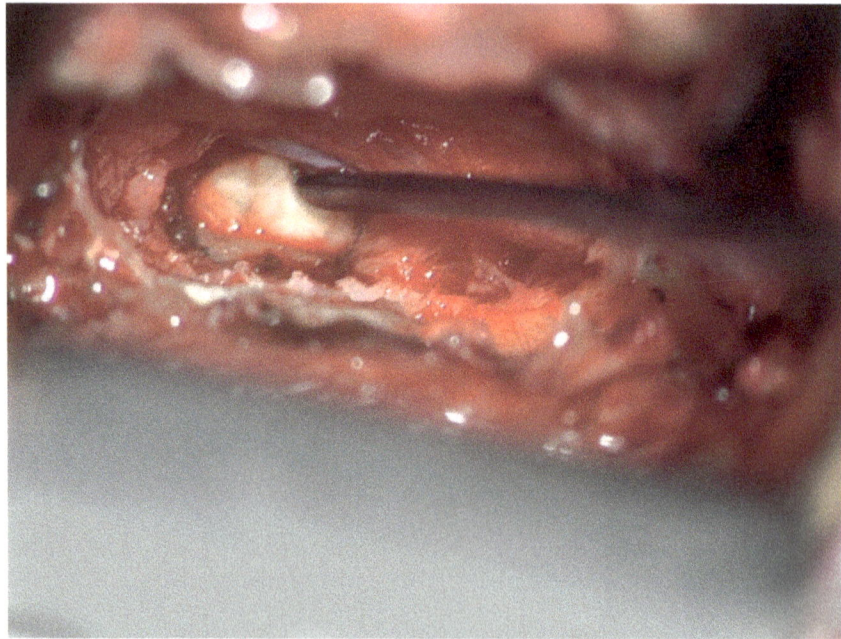

Fig. 3.90: Gently retract the nerve root with a small dissector

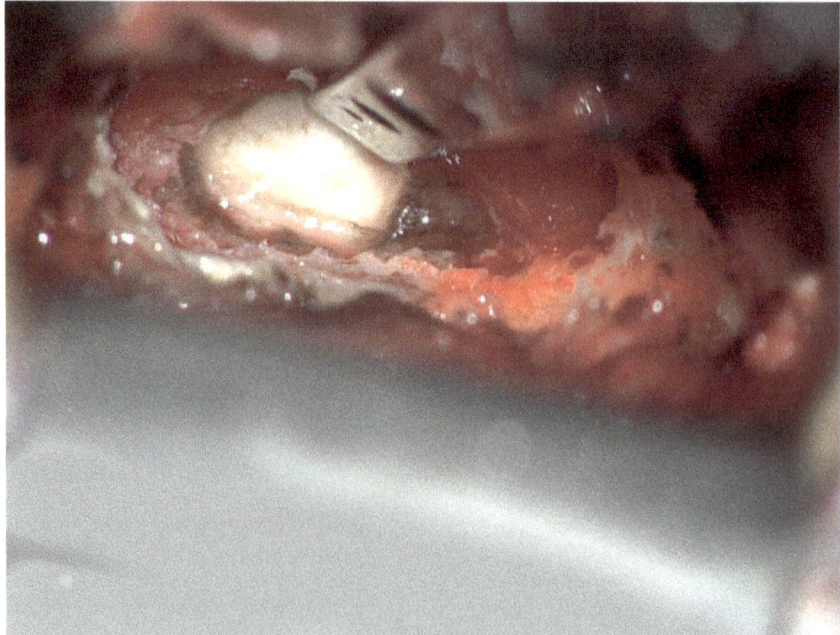

Fig. 3.91: Secure the nerve root with a retractor and expose the bulging annulus. This will give a good assessment of the ventral compression

Operative Techniques with Case Examples | 67

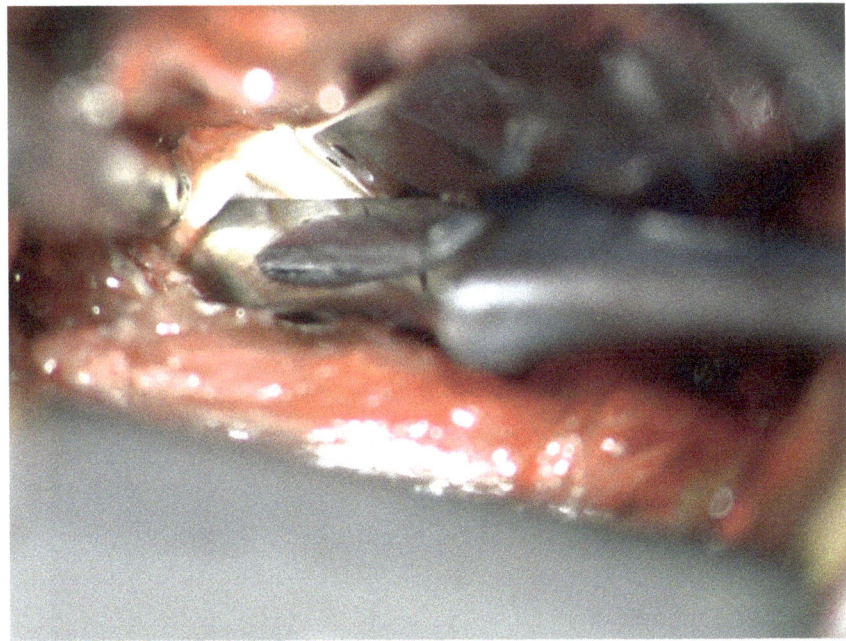

Fig. 3.92: Cut the annulus with No. 11 blade knife

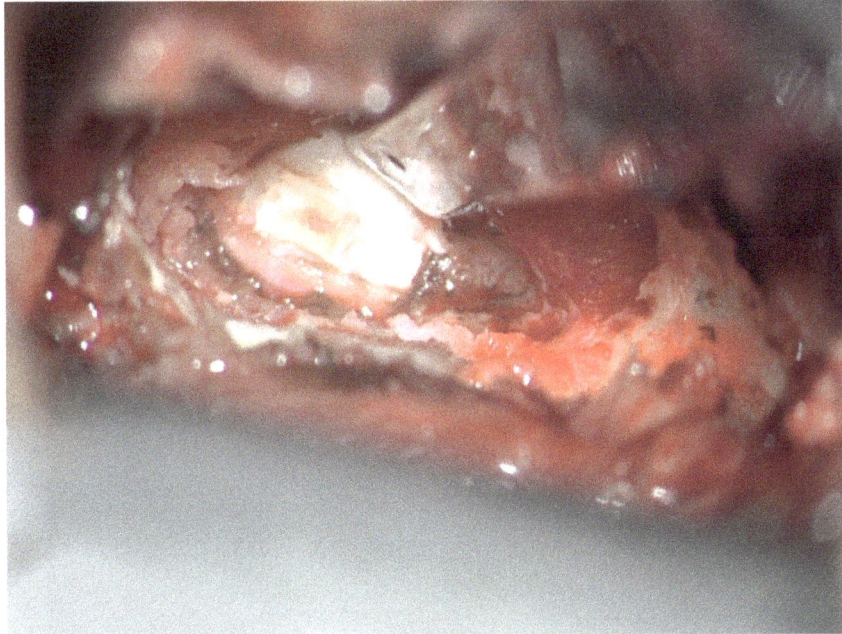

Fig. 3.93: Press the annulus with the base of nerve root retractor

Discectomy done methodically **(Figs 3.94 to 3.98)**. Intradiscal disc is removed with angled disc punches **(Figs 3.99 to 3.102)**. Ligamentum flavum is removed **(Figs 3.103 and 3.104)**. The laxity of the nerve root confirms good discectomy **(Fig. 3.105)**. Entire length of the nerve root should be inspected and a nerve root probe is inserted in the foramen to ensure the free nerve root **(Figs 3.106 and 3.107)**.

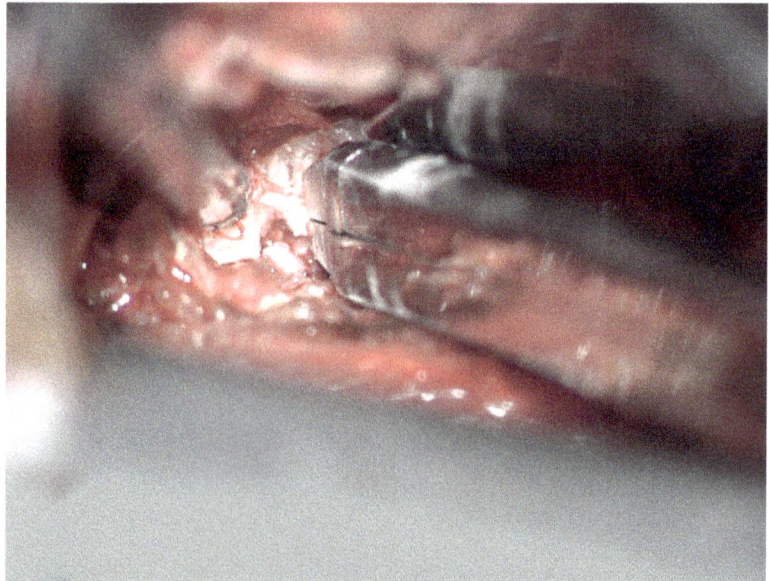

Fig. 3.94: Remove the extruded disc material

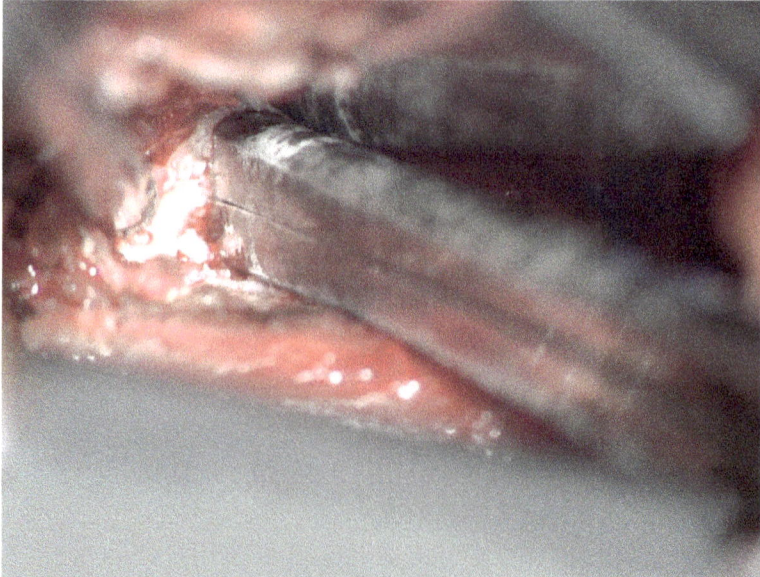

Fig. 3.95: Insert the disc punch gently in the disc space. Do not exert pressure

Operative Techniques with Case Examples | 69

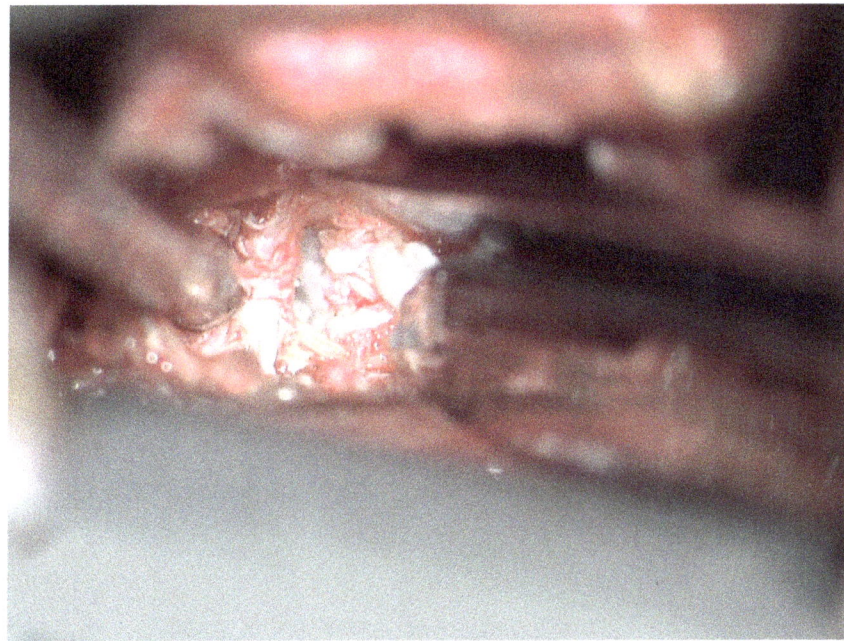

Fig. 3.96: Remove the free disc material from the disc space. The annulus thus gets lax further

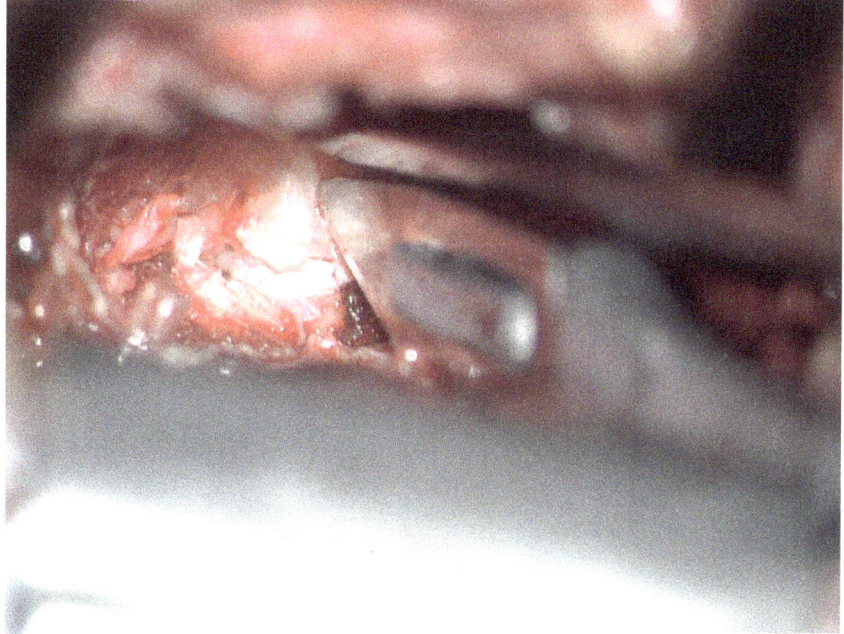

Fig. 3.97: Now, retract the nerve root further and cut the annulus further medially

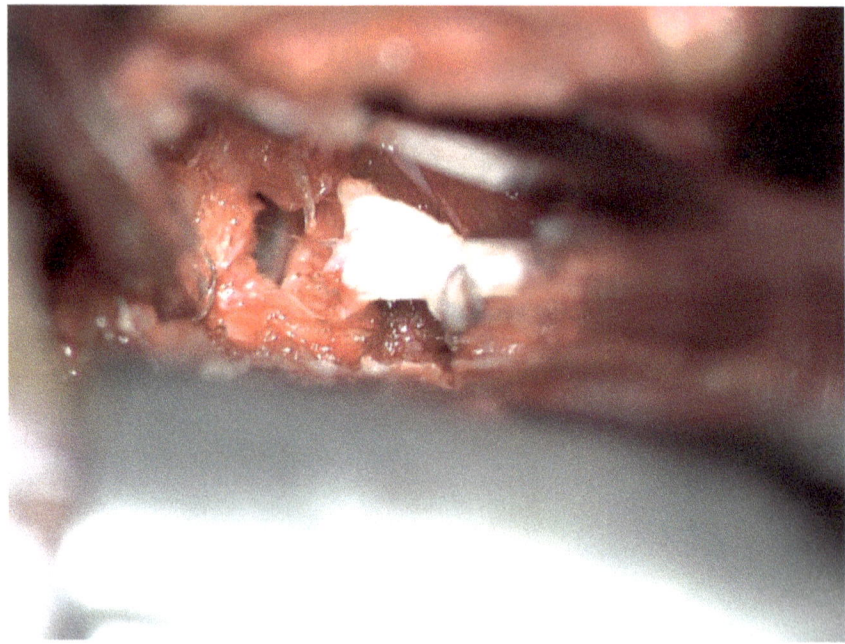

Fig. 3.98: Remove the bulging annulus and the disc material underneath

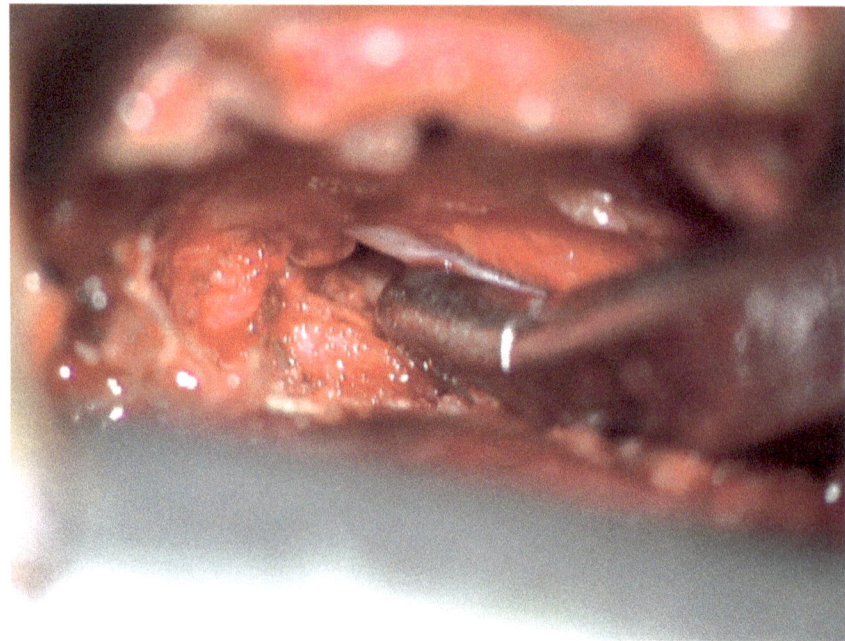

Fig. 3.99: Forward angled disc punch is now used to enter the disc space

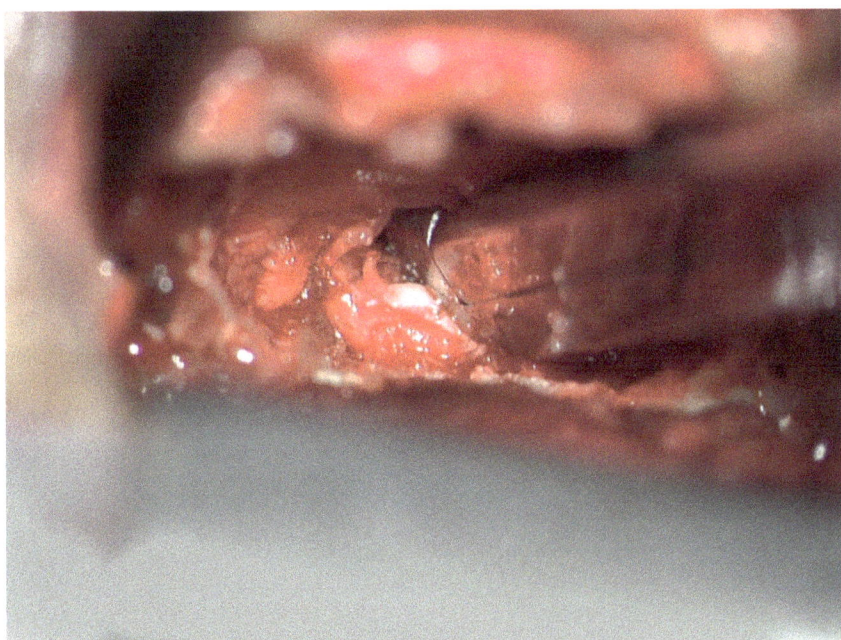

Fig. 3.100: Enter the tip gently in the disc space and search for free disc material that is below the annulus on the opposite site

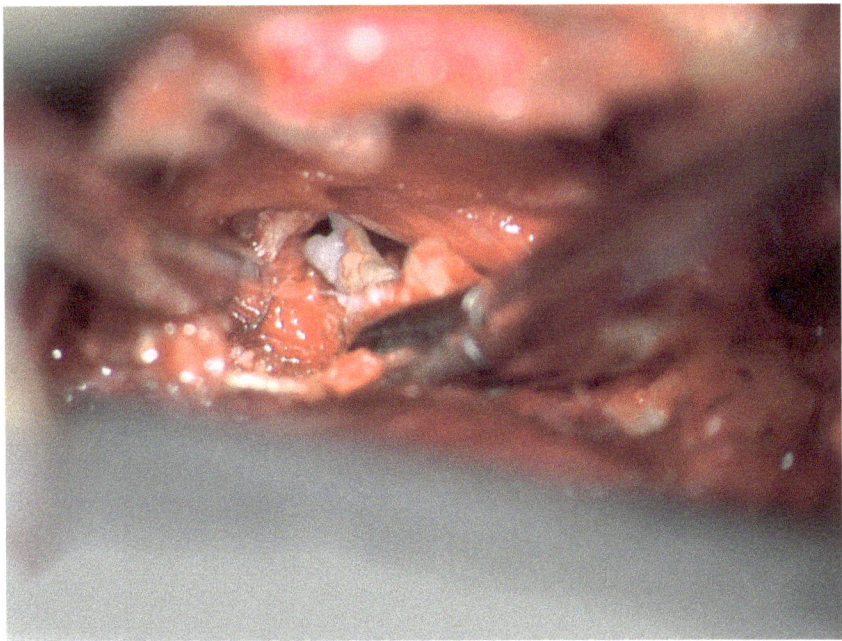

Fig. 3.101: 'Fish out' the free disc material gently

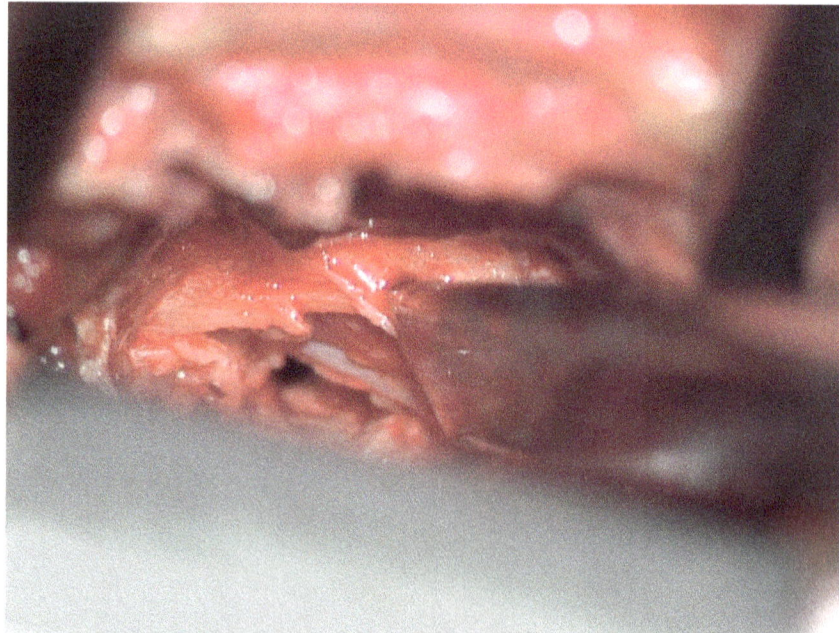

Fig. 3.102: Medial part of ligamentum flavum if needed can be removed

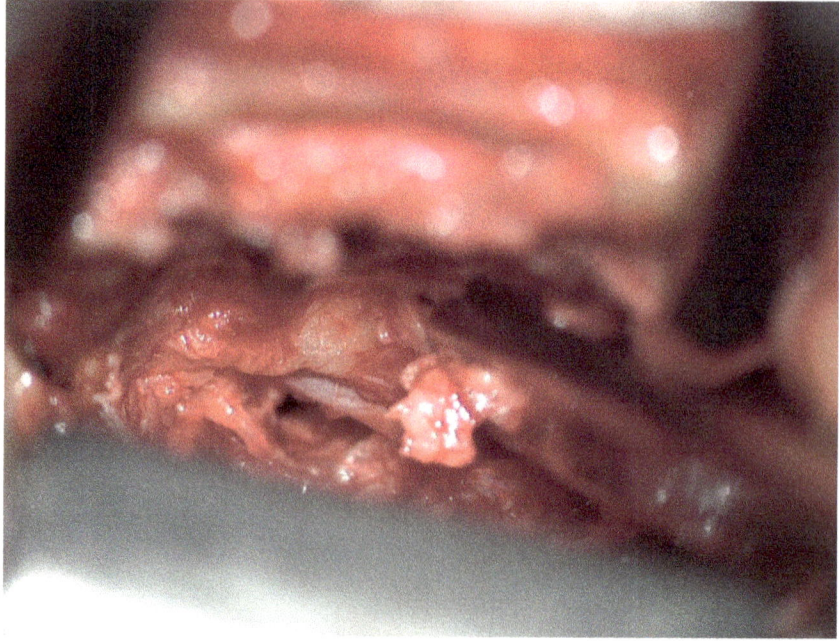

Fig. 3.103: This step is to just confirm a good lateral canal decompression

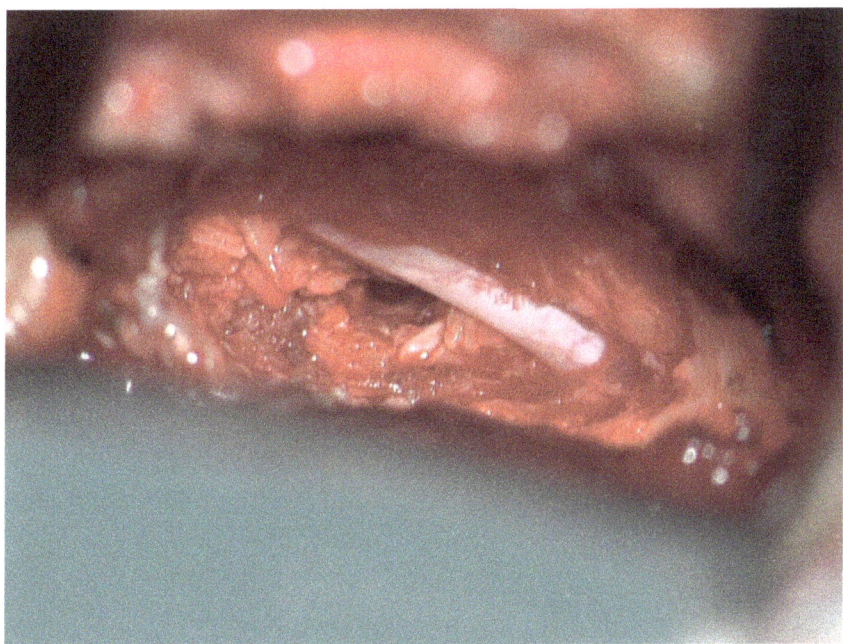

Fig. 3.104: Entire length of the nerve root is lax now

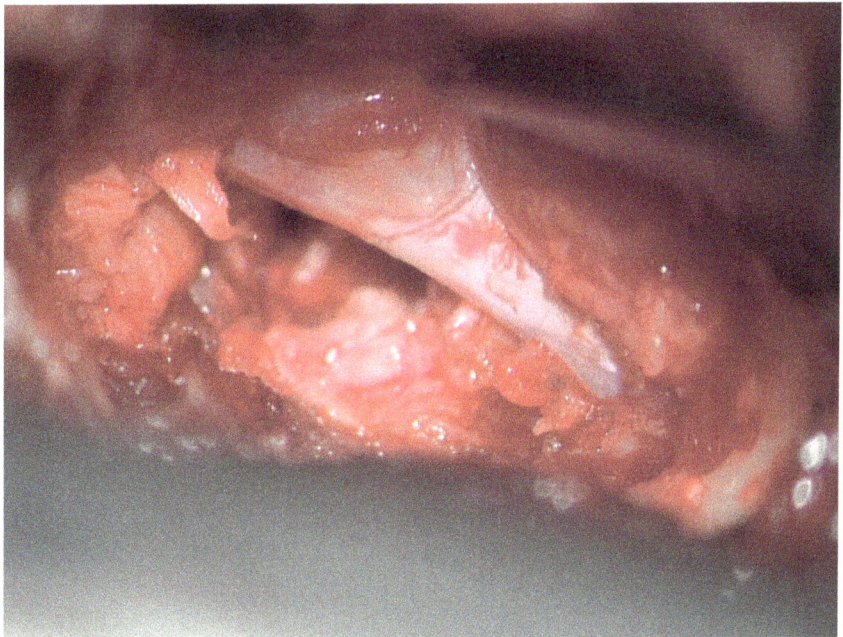

Fig. 3.105: Lax nerve root moves after satisfactory decompression and visible under microscope

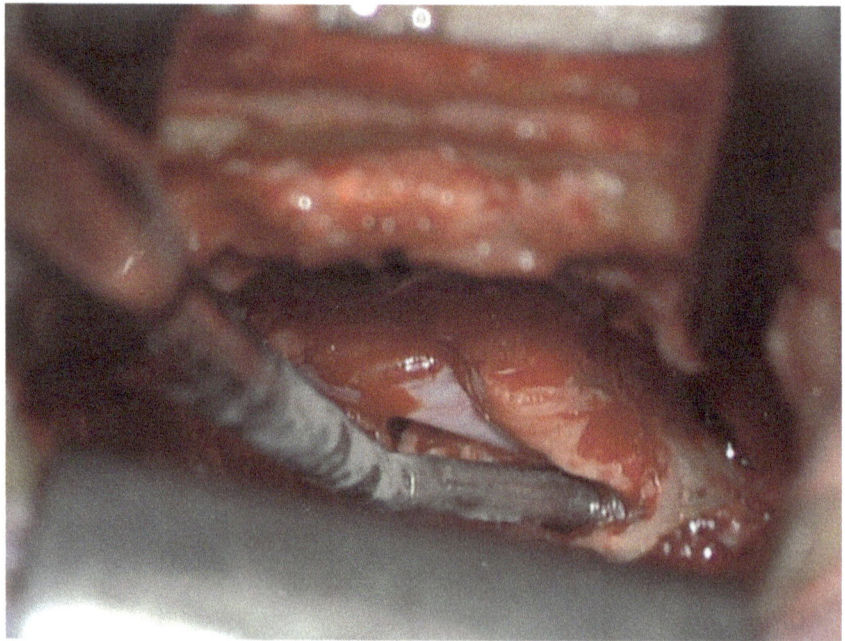

Fig. 3.106: Root canal probe is now entered through the canal

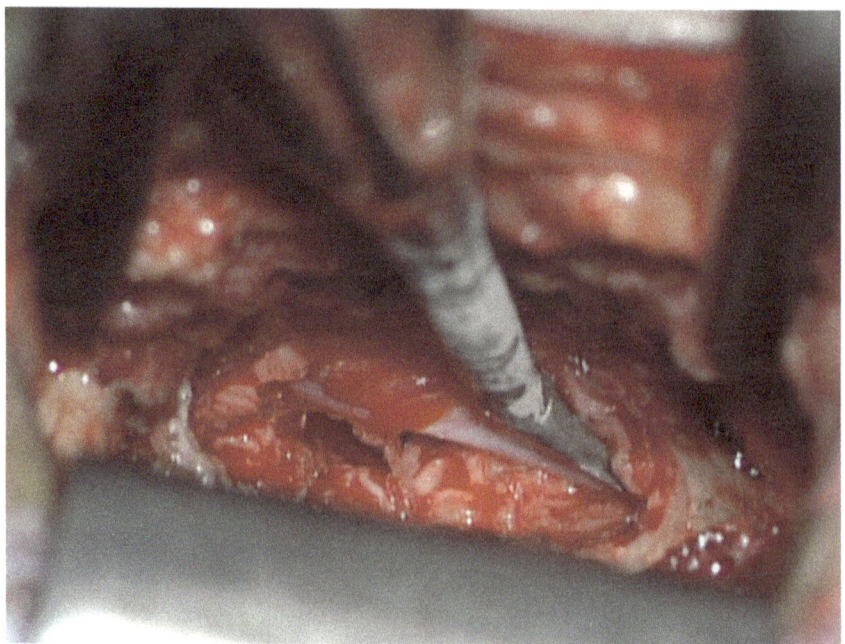

Fig. 3.107: Free entry of the probe in the canal confirms distal decompression

Lateral Disc Prolapse—Upper Level

Case example: Upper level lumbar disc prolapses are less encountered. The canal is narrower and nerve roots are vertical in comparison to lower level. The interlaminar space is also narrower. Often one has to perform medial facetectomy and partial laminotomy in these cases while discectomy. Below is a case example of L_2/L_3 posterolateral large disc prolapse presenting on right side.

Clinical status: Right side L_3 dermatomal sensory loss, absent knee jerk and pain **(Figs 3.108 and 3.109)**.

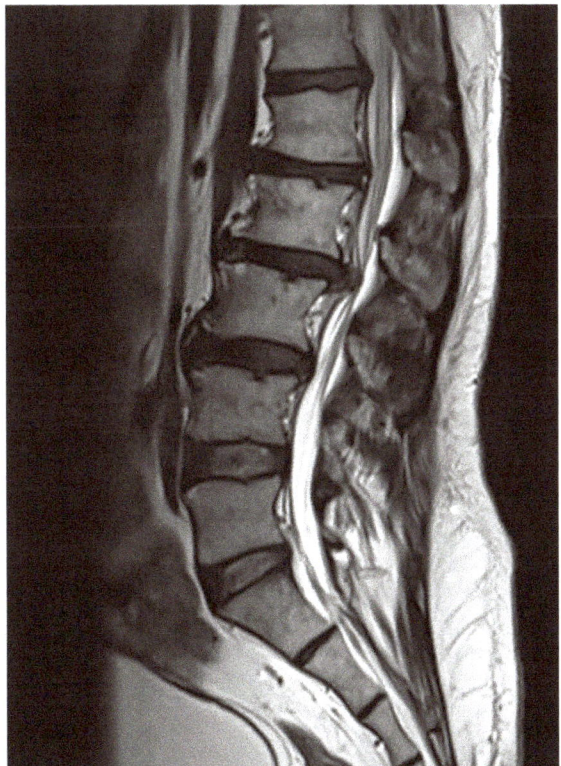

Fig. 3.108: MRI sagittal view showing L_2/L_3 disc prolapse with cauda equina compression

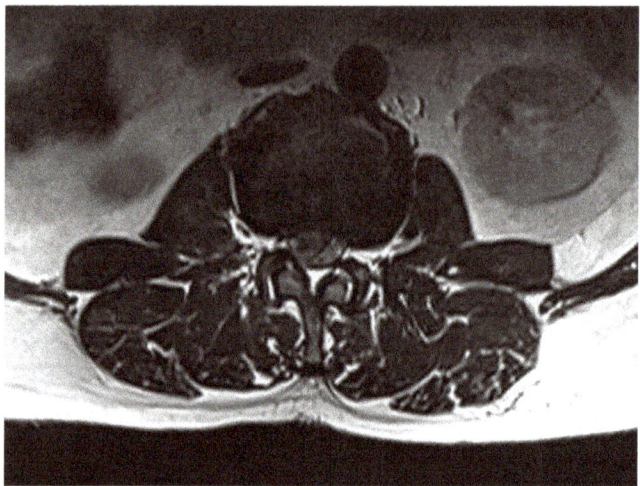

Fig. 3.109: MRI axial view showing the large disc prolapse on right side with dural compression

Operative Procedure (Fig. 110A)

Step 1-Exposure of interlaminar space: The interlaminar space is exposed as detailed in previous chapter. The lamina and facet joints are thicker and narrower and hence a very narrow a interlaminar space **(Fig. 3.110B)**. Even in the best possible position the interspinous distance is not much wide

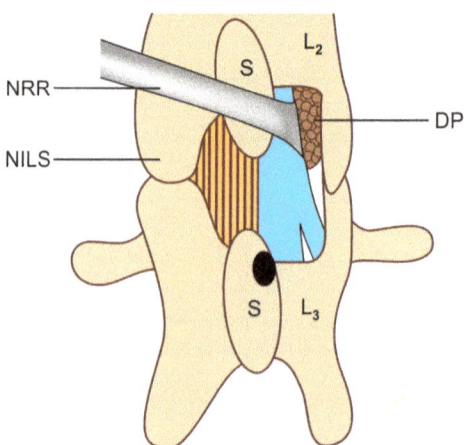

Fig. 3.110A
Abbreviations: DP, disc prolapse; L, lamina; NILS, narrow interlaminar space; NRR, nerve root retractor; S, spinous process

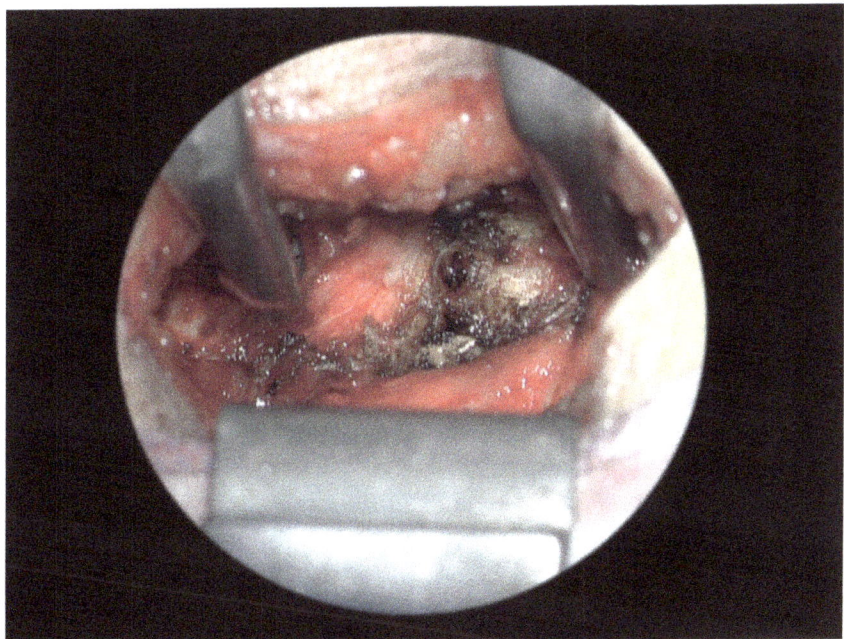

Fig. 3.110B: Interlaminar space exposed. The space is narrow at the upper level especially at L_{1-2} and L_{2-3}

compared to lower level. I usually avoid too much of flexion while positioning the patient for upper levels since the canal is narrower and cauda equina is compromised significantly in these cases. This, in fact, reduces the chance of neurological deficit due to overstretching.

Step 2-Lateral canal decompression and exposing disc: As described earlier, a good lateral canal decompression should be done. Since the canal is narrow and the contents are crowded, drilling and excision of bone should be meticulous **(Fig. 3.111)**. Since the nerve roots are vertical at the upper level, we may not be visualizing the nerve root as easy as in the lower level. Dura will be seen bulging and need to be retracted gently to reach the disc space **(Figs 3.112 and 3.113)**.

Step 3-Discectomy: Cauterize the epidural bleeders. Incise the annulus and pull out the disc fragments from under the annulus by gently pushing the annulus down by the retractor blade **(Figs 3.114 to 3.116)**. Annulus will become lax and the dura may look lax too **(Fig. 3.117)**. Now at this stage, always check the MRI findings and do no hesitate to search further medially and inside the disc space for free fragments **(Fig. 3.118)**. Fish out all free fragments until satisfactory discectomy and decompression of nerve root is achieved **(Figs 3.119 to 3.121)**. Movement of dural sleeve should be appreciated at the end of the procedure under magnification **(Fig. 3.122)**.

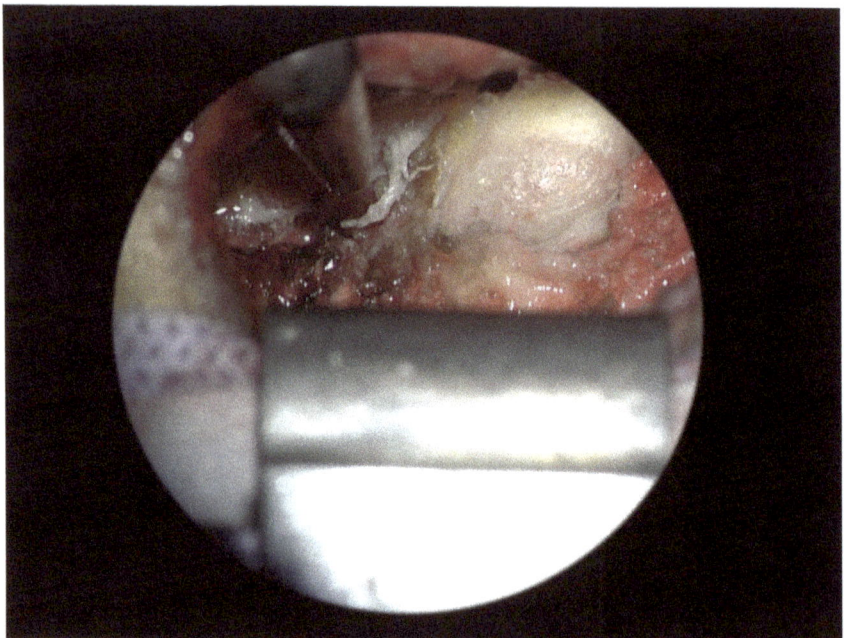

Fig. 3.111: Inferior one-third of lamina and medial one-third of the facet of upper vertebra drilled out. The pale yellow indicates the laminar area

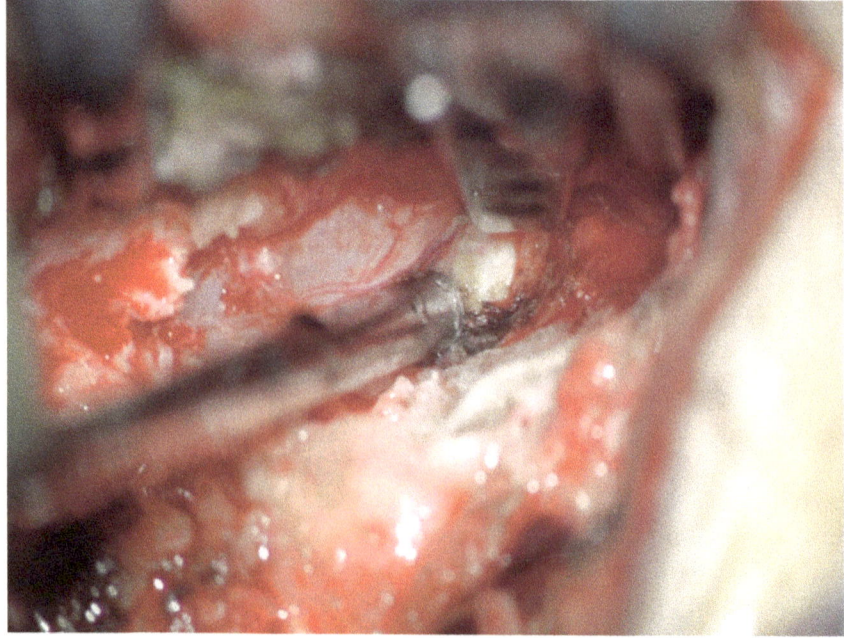

Fig. 3.112: Lateral canal deroofing done and the dura retracted to expose the disc space

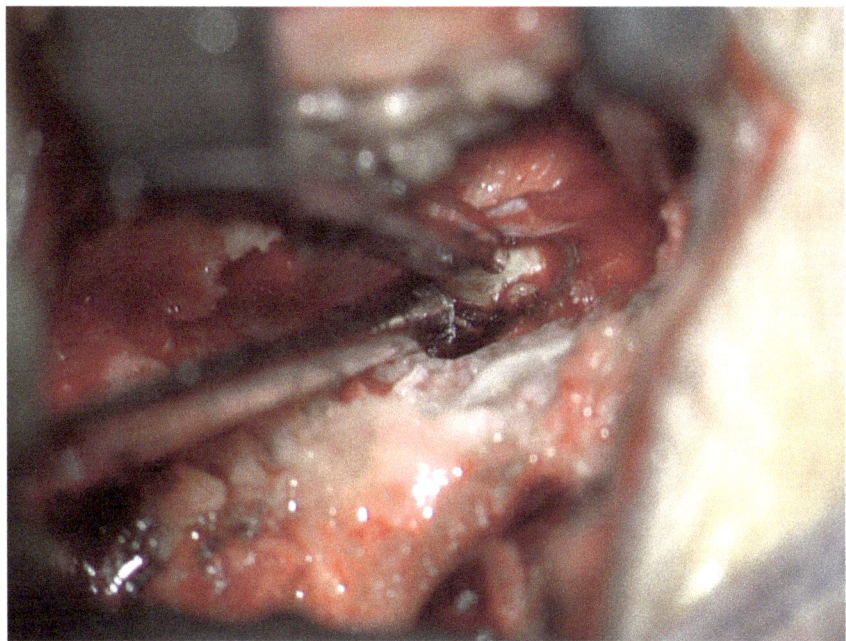

Fig. 3.113: Bulging annulus is well visualized. Epidural bleeders are coagulated

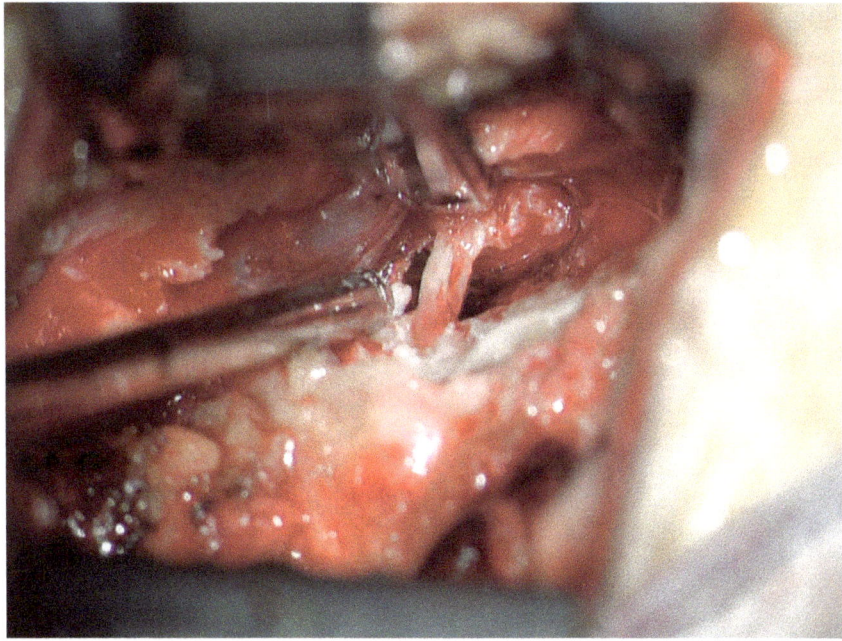

Fig. 3.114: Annulus is incised and disc material is exposed

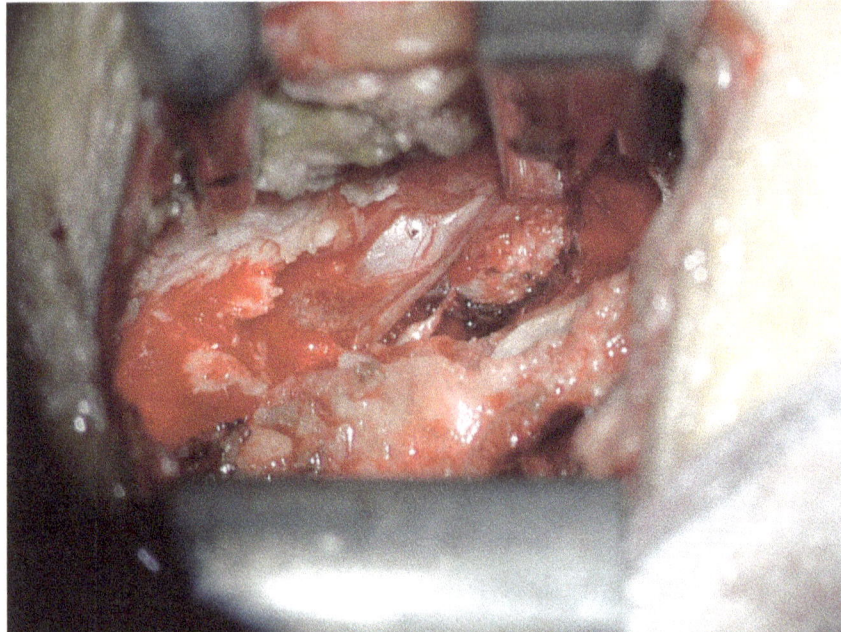

Fig. 3.115: Remove the disc material

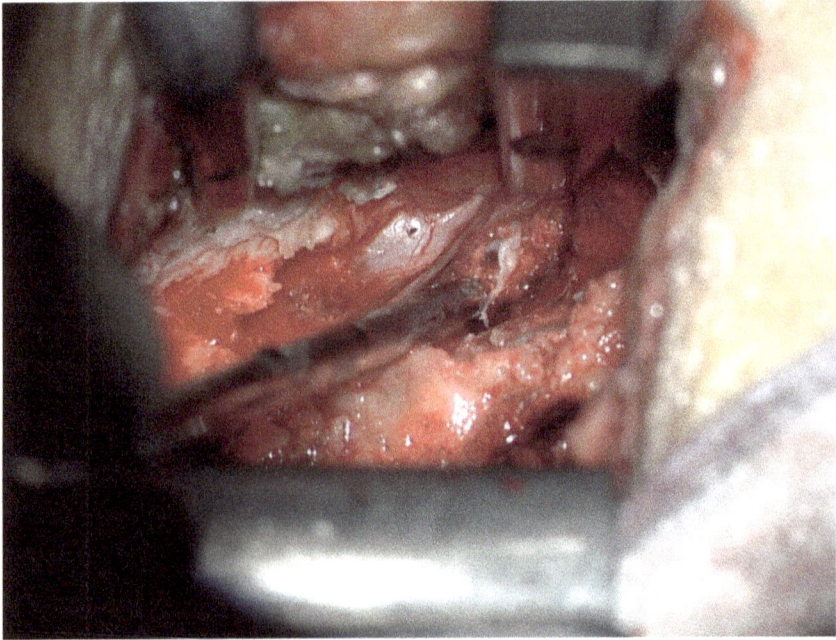

Fig. 3.116: Inspect the subannular region to expose more

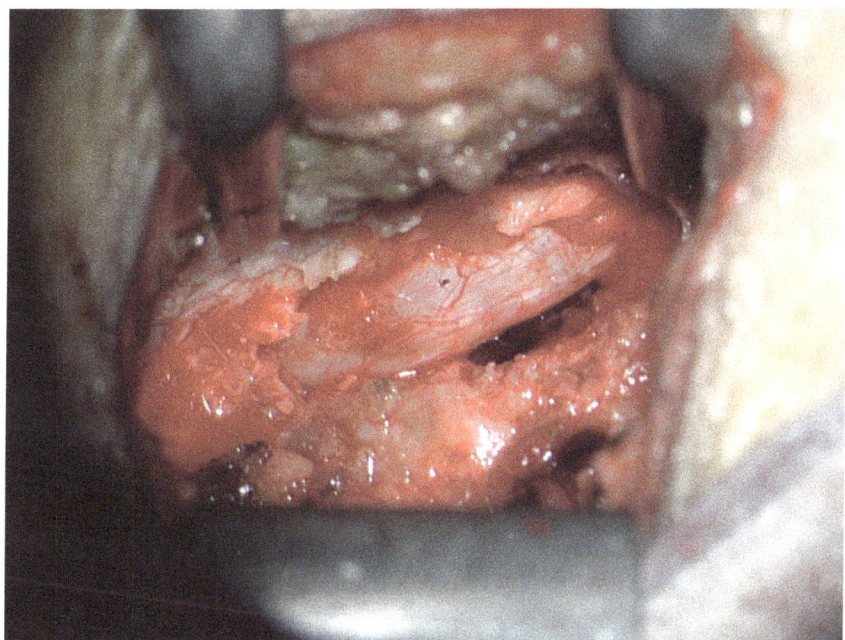

Fig. 3.117: Dura may lock lax here and the nerve root is not seen well as in the lower level. Correlate with MRI for further search

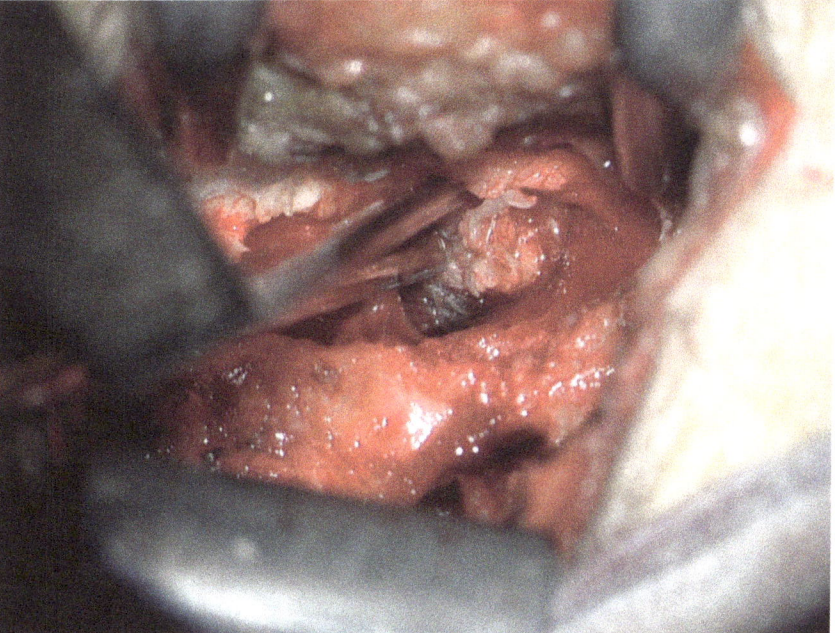

Fig. 3.118: Retracting the dura further and exposing more annulus medially allows further exploration in the disc space

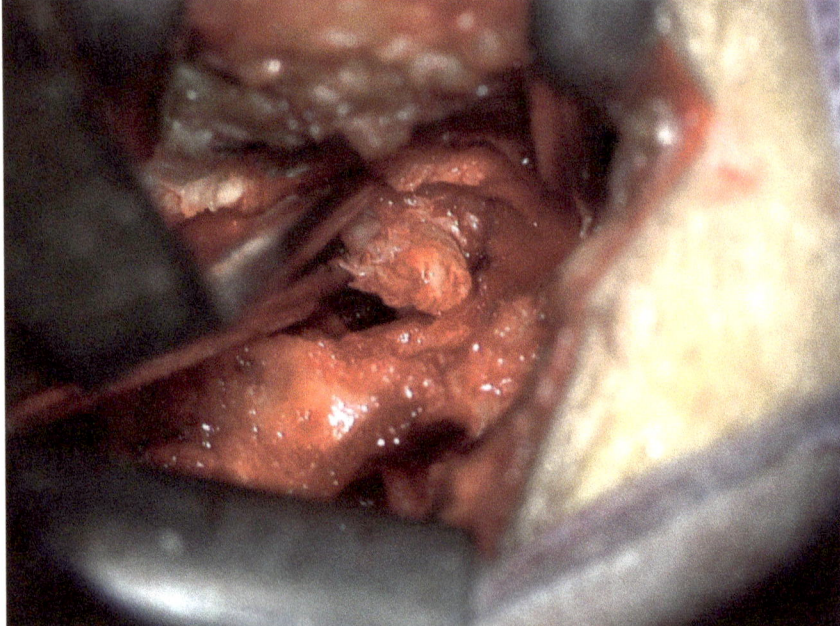

Fig. 3.119: Large subannular and intradiscal free fragment need to be 'fished out'

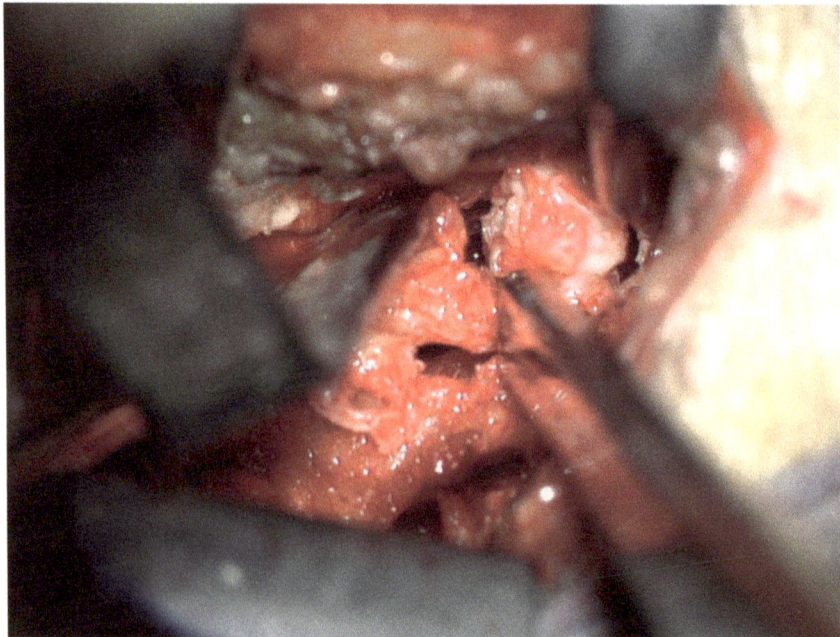

Fig. 3.120: Remove the fragments with disc punch until satisfactory nerve root and dural decompression is achieved

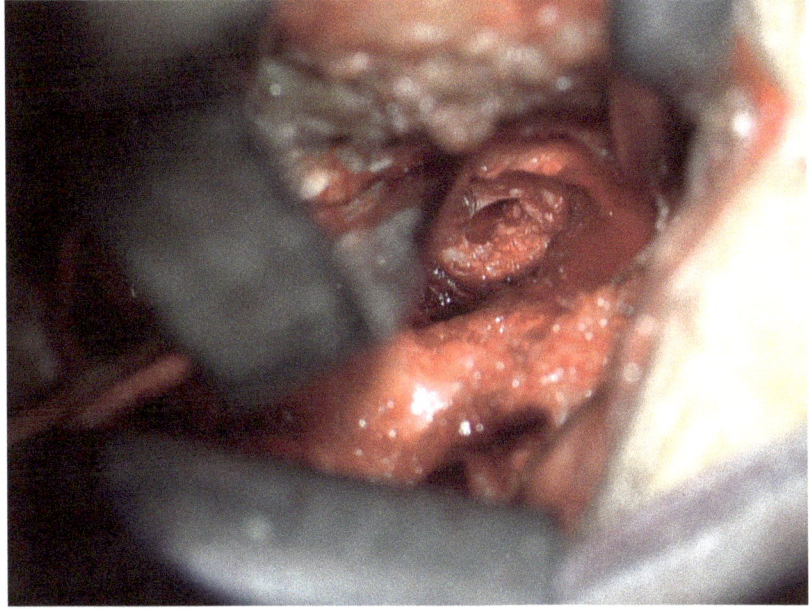

Fig. 3.121: Annular incision through which the intradiscal fragments removed

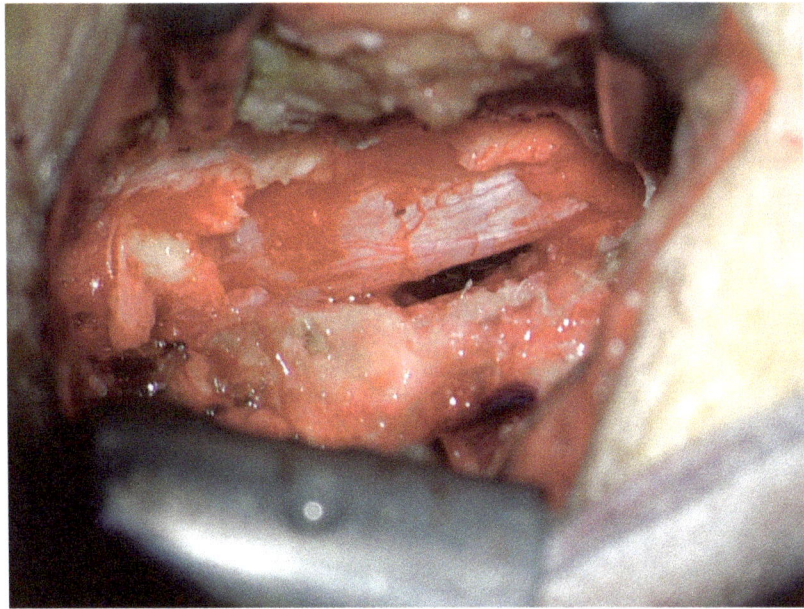

Fig. 3.122: Dural pulsation is seen well in magnification

MIGRATION

Inferior Migration of Large Fragments—Central and Lateral

Case example: L_5/S_1 large inferiorly migrated disc prolapse. Bilobed and centrolaterally placed at the level of disc and below.

Clinical status: Cauda equina syndrome with sciatica on right side **(Figs 3.123 to 3.125)**.

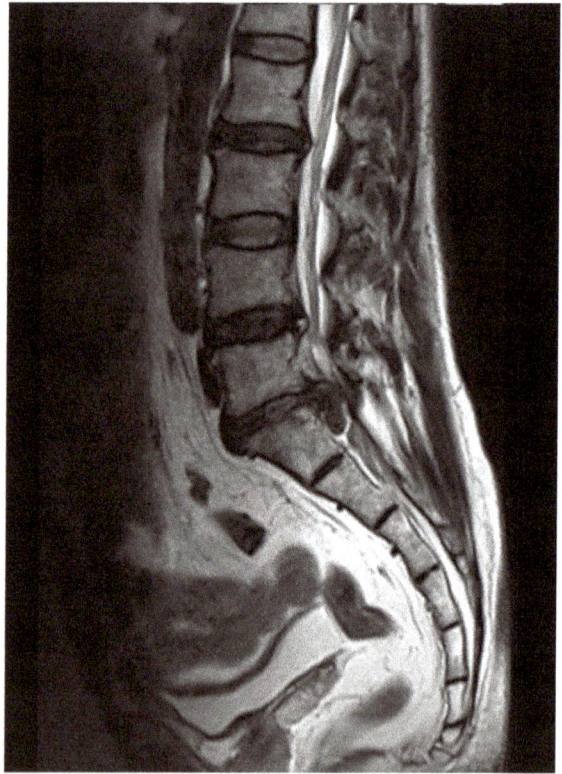

Fig. 3.123: MRI sagittal view showing a large disc prolapse at L_5/S_1 level migrating inferiorly. Bilobed disc fragments

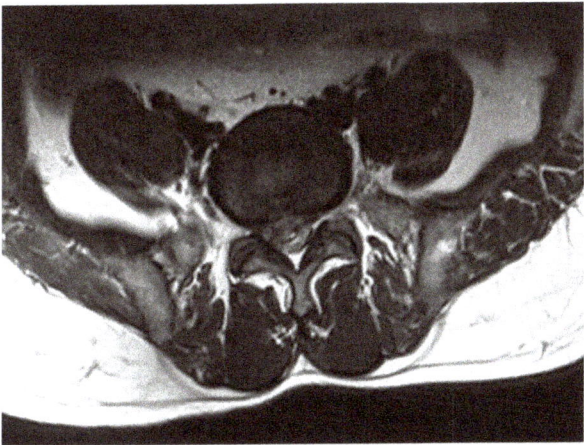

Fig. 3.124: MRI axial view showing a large disc prolapse at central and lateral region with severe canal stenosis

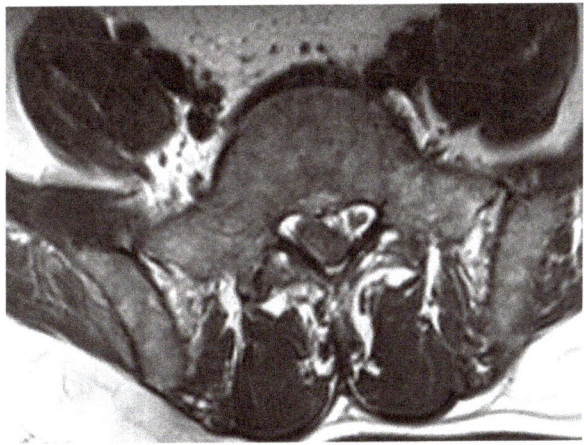

Fig. 3.125: MRI axial view showing inferiorly migrated fragment causing significant canal compromise laterally on the right side

Operative Procedure (Fig. 3.126A)

Step 1-Exposure of interlaminar epidural space: Since the disc prolapse is large in size with significant inferior migration adequate excision of sacral lamina is performed **(Fig. 3.126B)**. Medial facetectomy **(Fig. 3.127)** and excision of the inferior border of upper lamina (L_5) is done as detailed earlier. The ligamentum flavum is removed well to expose the large epidural space.

Step 2-Discectomy axillary approach: Epidural space is dissected to identify the nerve root **(Fig. 3.128)**. The axillary region of S_1 nerve root is inspected

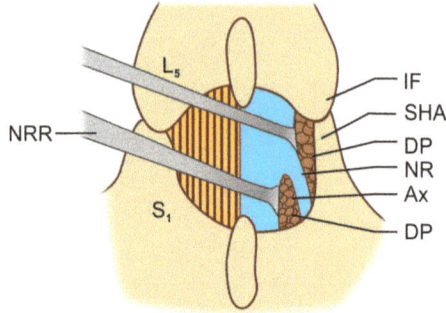

Fig. 3.126A
Abbreviations: Ax, axillary approach; DP, disc prolapse; IF, Inferior facet; NR, nerve root; SHA, shoulder approach

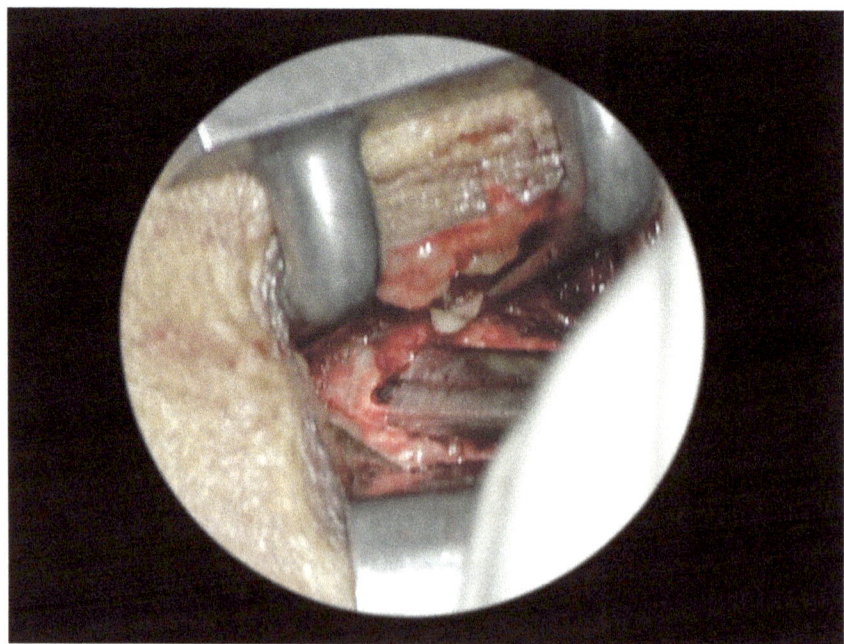

Fig. 3.126B: Superior border of sacral lamina is excised

Operative Techniques with Case Examples | 87

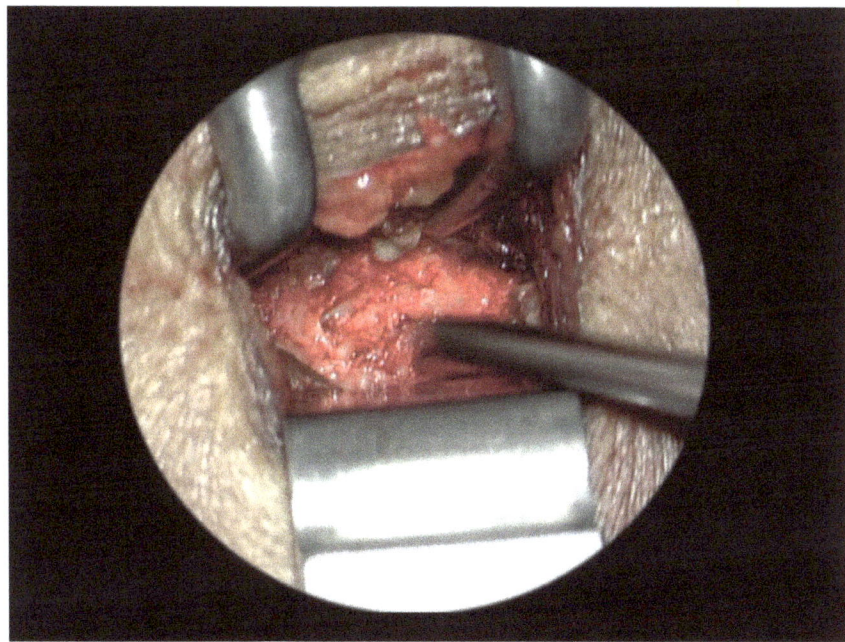

Fig. 3.127: Medial facetectomy done and ligamentum flavum excised

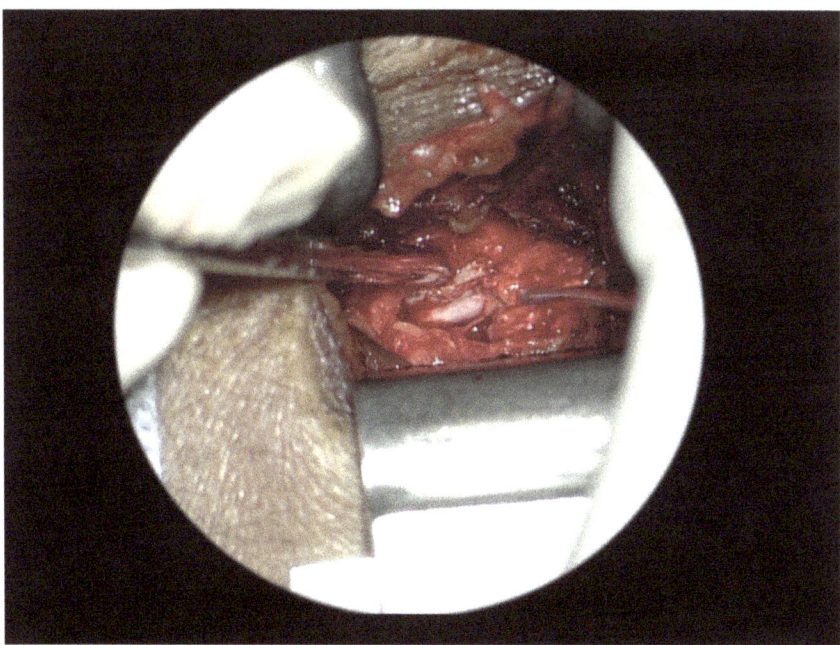

Fig. 3.128: Nerve root is identified

(medial to nerve root) **(Fig. 3.129)**. In this case, the degenerated fragments that have migrated inferiorly is seen easily **(Fig. 3.130)**. Fragments are hooked and removed **(Fig. 3.131)**. Further exploration done in the axillary region to remove all hidden large fragments **(Fig. 3.132 and 3.133)**. This decompresses cauda equina fibers at the sacral vertebral body level.

Step 3–Discectomy shoulder approach: Focus is then shifted to cephalad and lateral to the nerve root (shoulder) at the disc level. Nerve root is retracted and bulging annulus exposed **(Fig. 3.134)**. Extruded disc fragments and free fragments inside the disc space is then removed as detailed in previous cases **(Fig. 3.135)**. This completes the process of satisfactory removal of pathological disc fragments and finally nerve root is decompressed well.

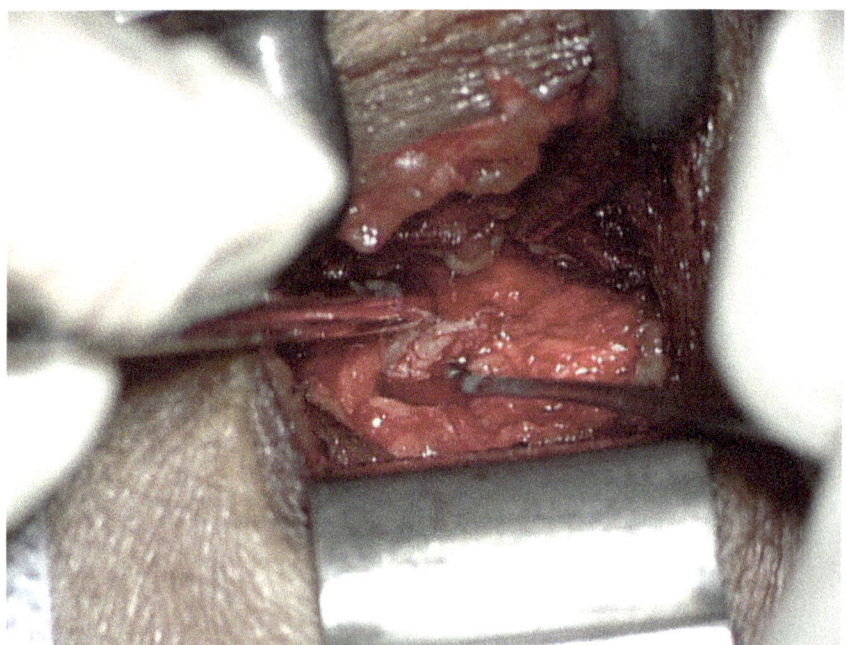

Fig. 3.129: Dissection carried medial to the nerve root through axillary approach

Operative Techniques with Case Examples

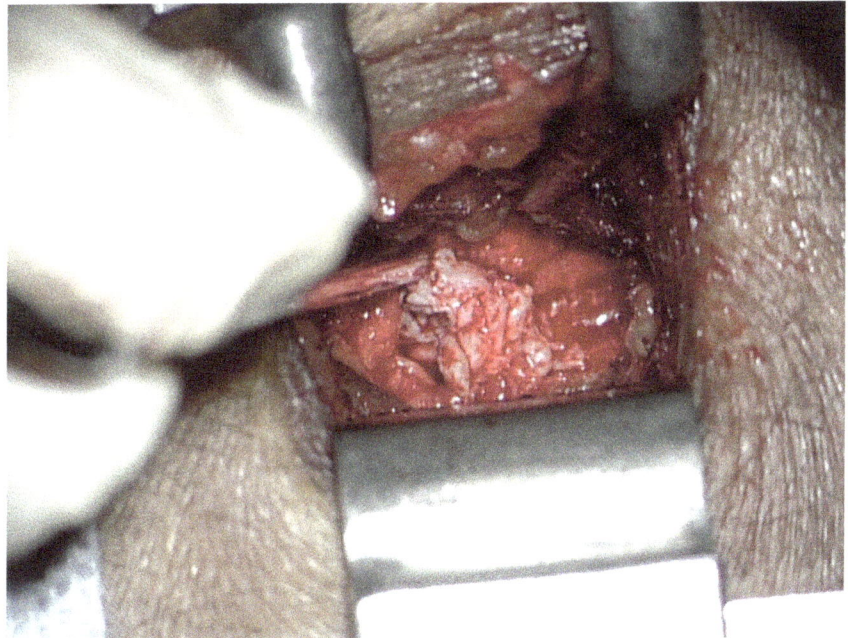

Fig. 3.130: Large inferiorly disc material seen easily

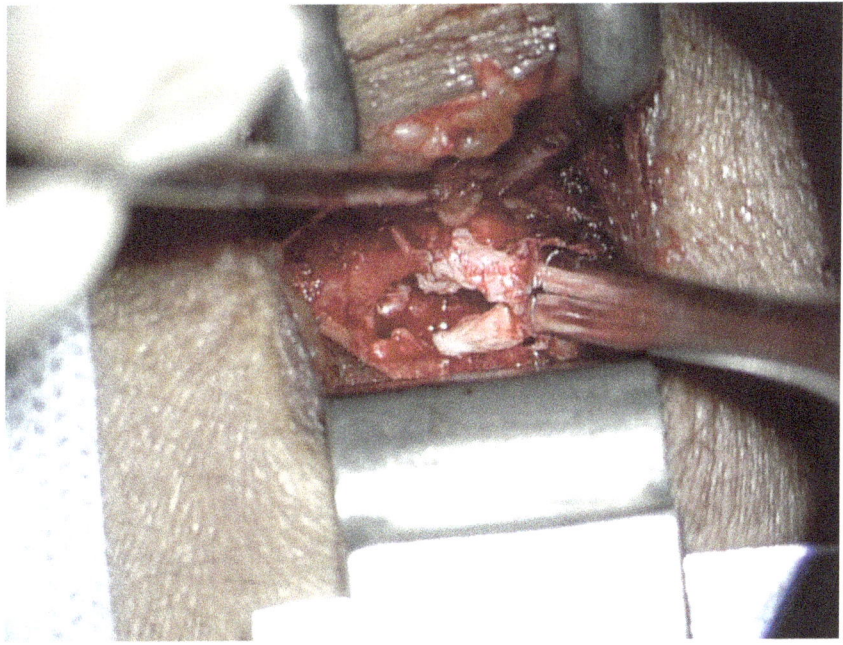

Fig. 3.131: Disc materials are removed

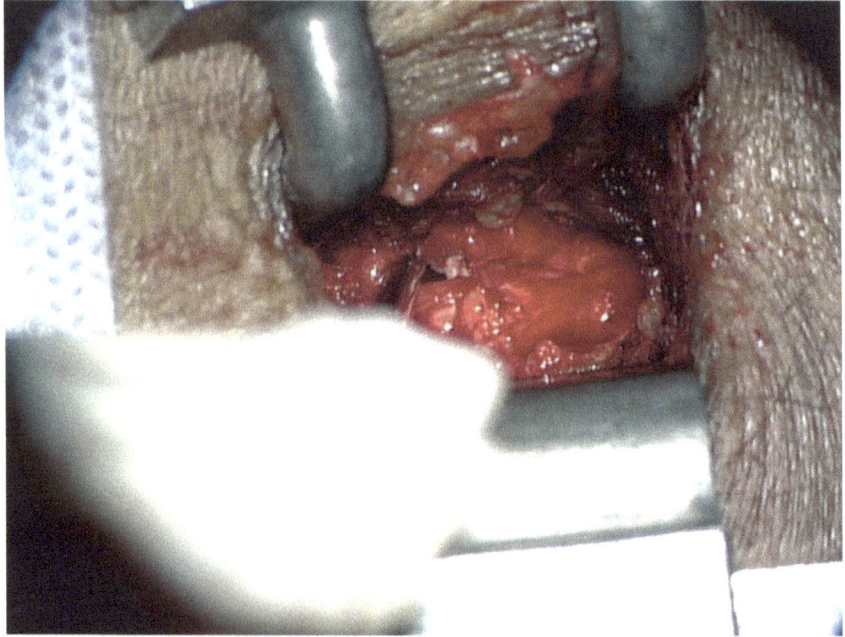

Fig. 3.132: Further dissection in the axillary region inferiorly exposes more fragments

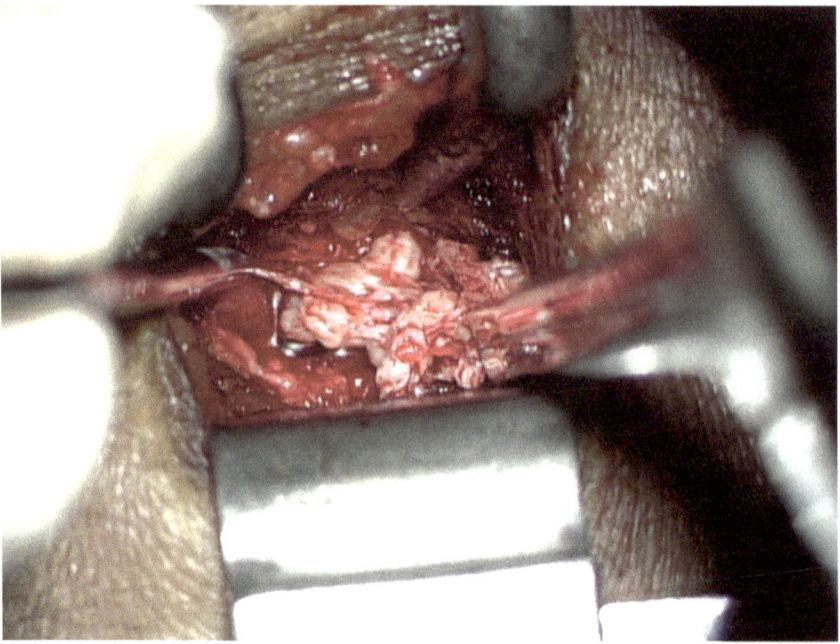

Fig. 3.133: All disc materials are removed

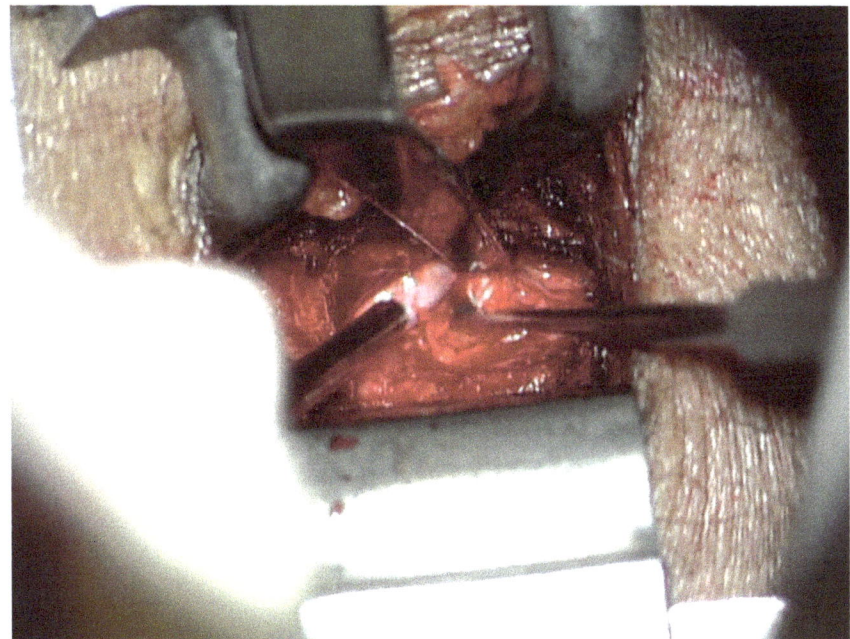

Fig. 3.134: Now nerve root is retracted above at the shoulder region medially

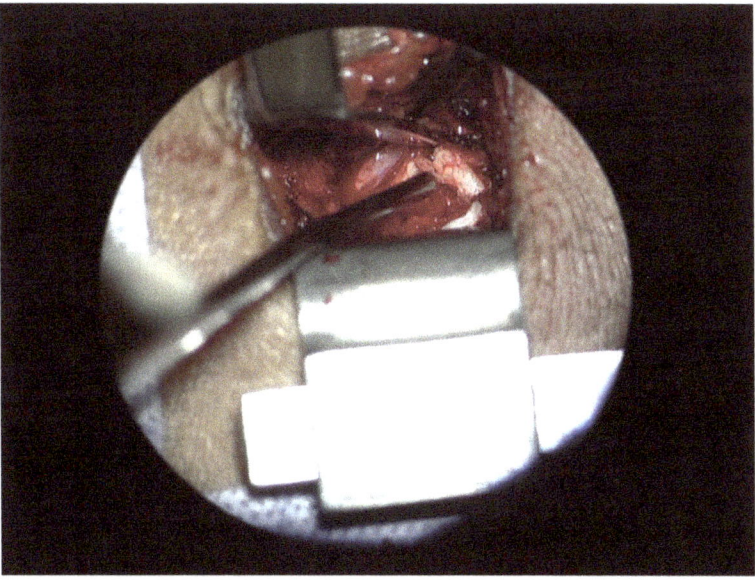

Fig. 3.135: Large disc materials at disc level is also removed

Inferior Migration—Central

Case example: L_5/S_1 disc prolapse and inferior migration in centrolateral position.

Clinical status: Sciatica right side **(Figs 3.136 and 3.137)**.

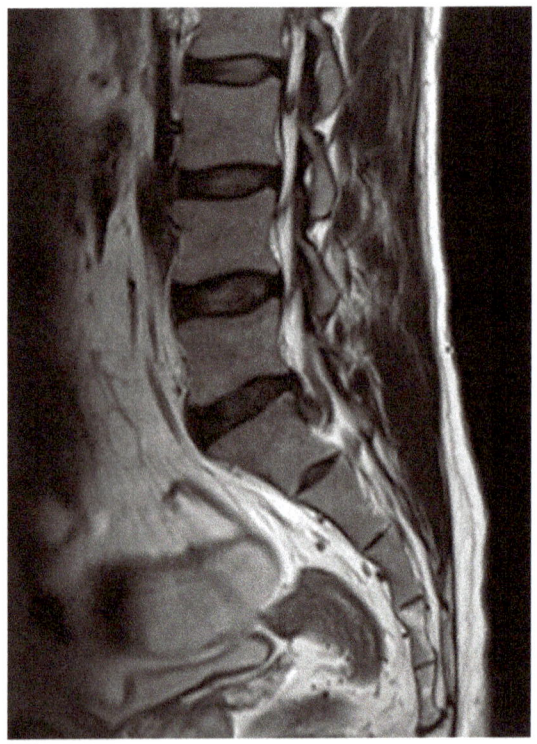

Fig. 3.136: MRI sagittal view showing disc prolapse at L_5/S_1 disc level. The disc fragment seen migrated inferiorly

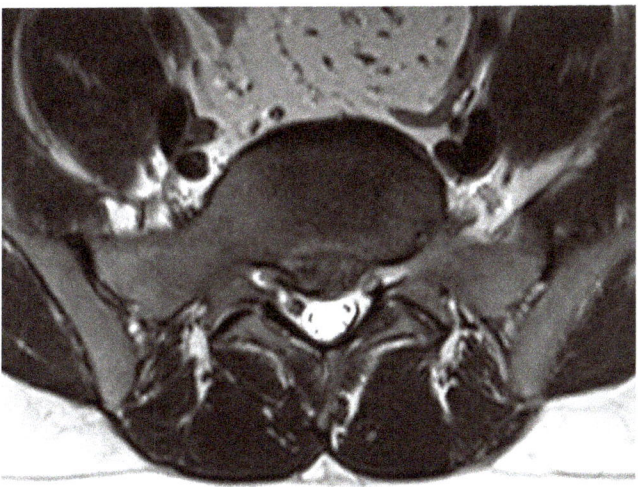

Fig. 3.137: MRI axial view showing migrated disc fragments at central

Operative Procedure (Fig. 138A)

Step 1-Excision of superior half of inferior lamina (S_1): Whenever the disc fragments are seen migrated inferiorly adequate exposure needs to be achieved by excising the superior half of the inferior lamina. This bony removal provides excellent visualization of areas inferior to disc space level. Using Kerrison punch, adequate lamina of sacral bone excised in this case **(Figs 3.138B and 3.139)**.

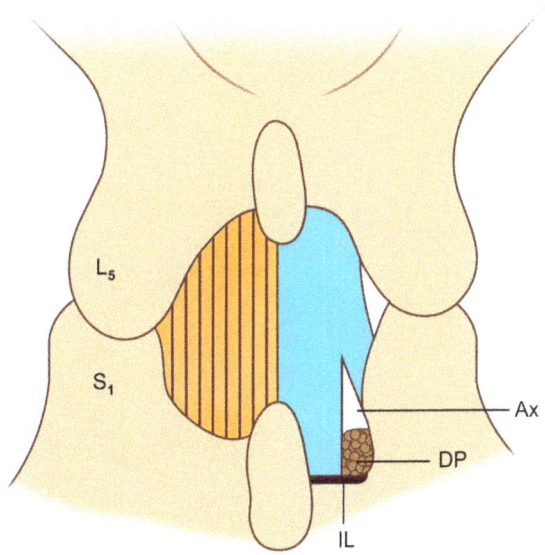

Fig. 3.138A
Abbreviations: Ax, axillary approach; DP, disc prolapse; IL, inferior lamina

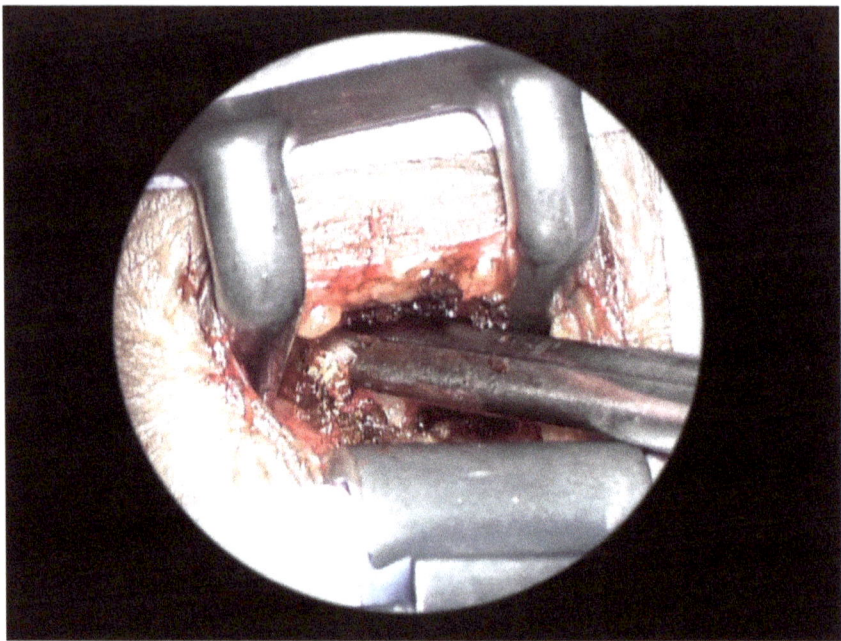

Fig. 3.138B: Excision of superior edge of sacral lamina

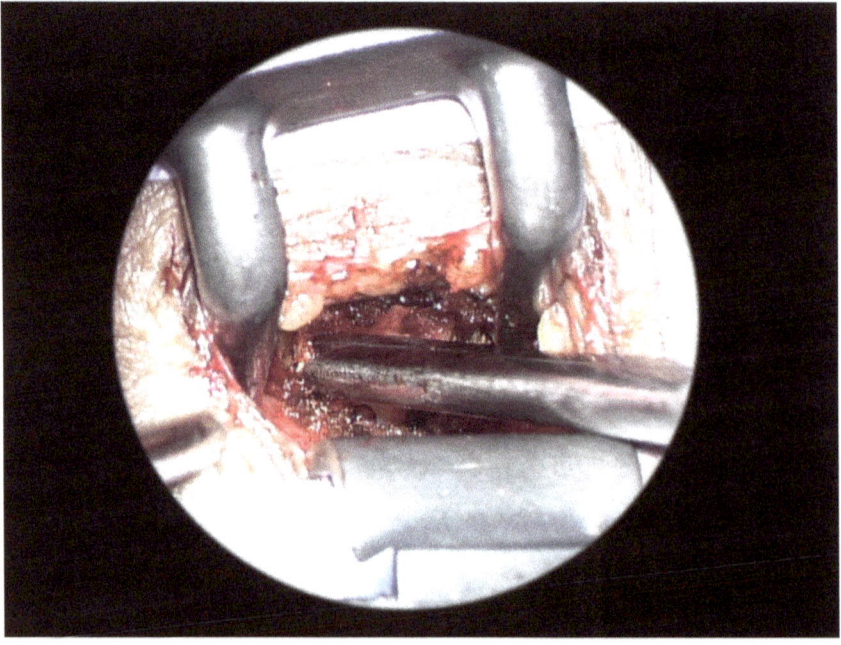

Fig. 3.139: Number 3 Kerrison punches are used

Step 2-Excision of ligamentum flavum: Ligamentum flavum removed as detailed earlier **(Fig. 3.140)**.

Step 3-Exploration for inferiorly migrated fragment: The epidural space dissected meticulously, fat lobules retracted to identify the nerve root. Then just below and medial to the L_5 nerve root, axillary region explored. Disc fragments seen at axially region **(Fig. 3.141)**.

Step 4-Discectomy: The disc fragments removed in piecemeal **(Fig. 3.142)**. Further exploration below the dura at lower level helped in identifying more fragments that migrated down **(Figs 3.143 and 3.144)**. Finally, the nerve roots and dura decompressed well.

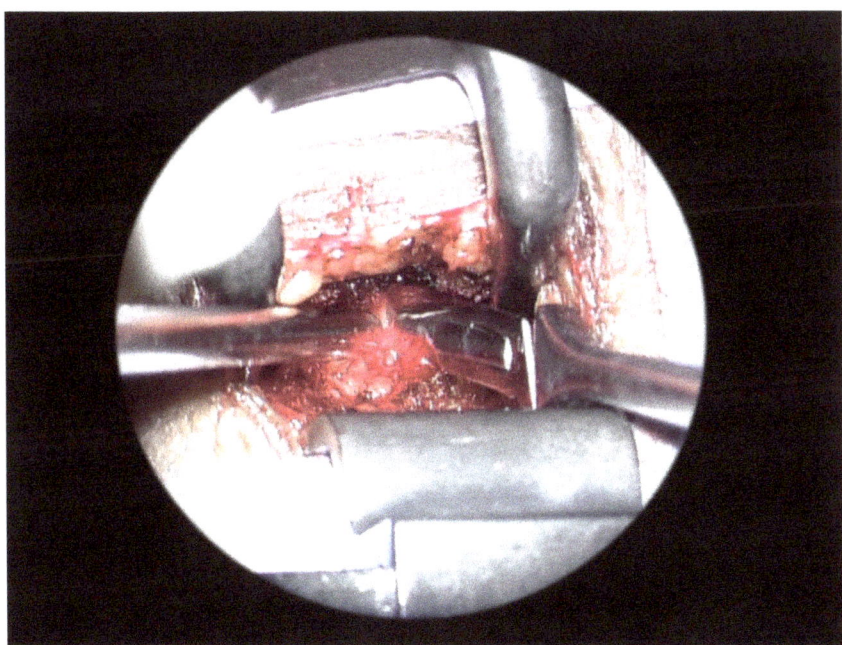

Fig. 3.140: Ligamentum flavum is incised and removed

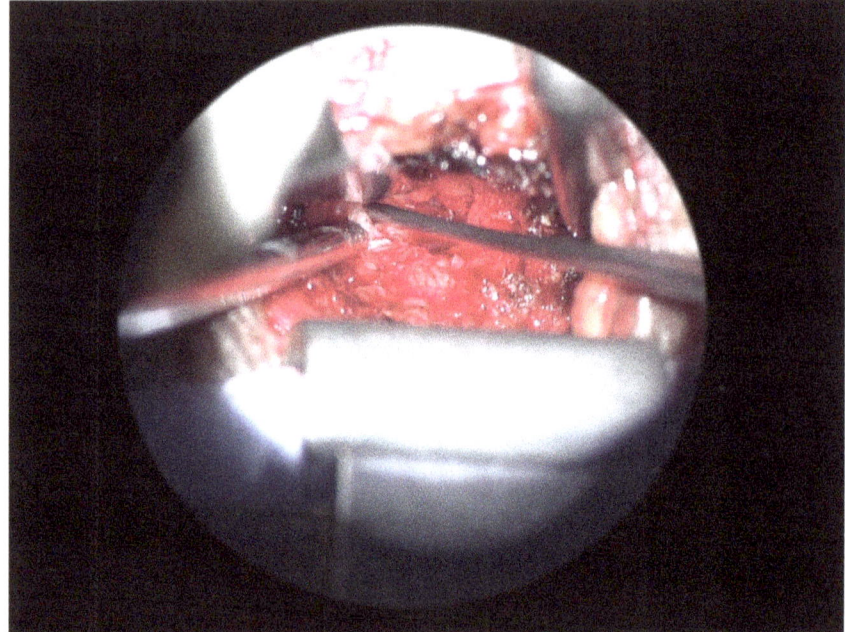

Fig. 3.141: Axillary region of the nerve root is probed

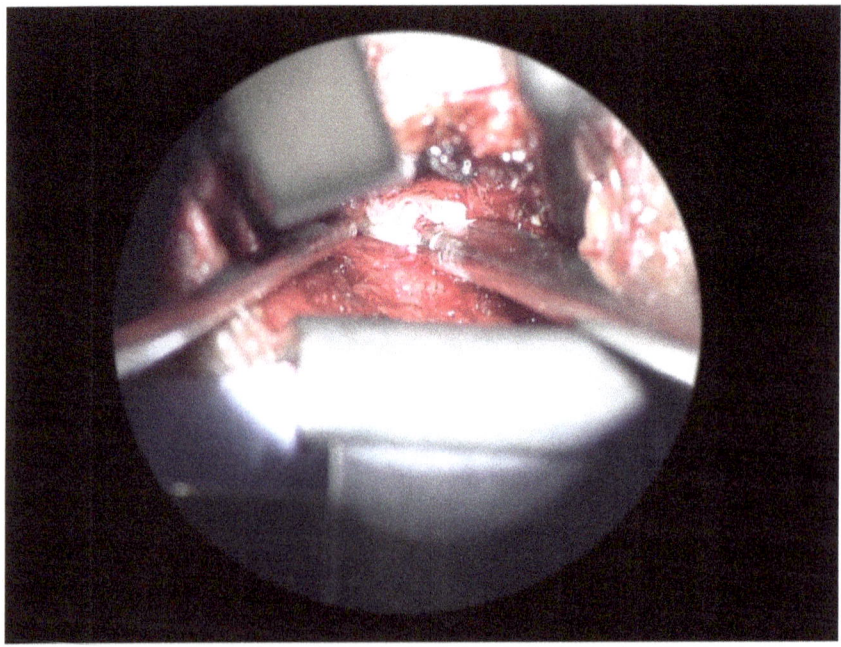

Fig. 3.142: Inferiorly migrated disc material removed

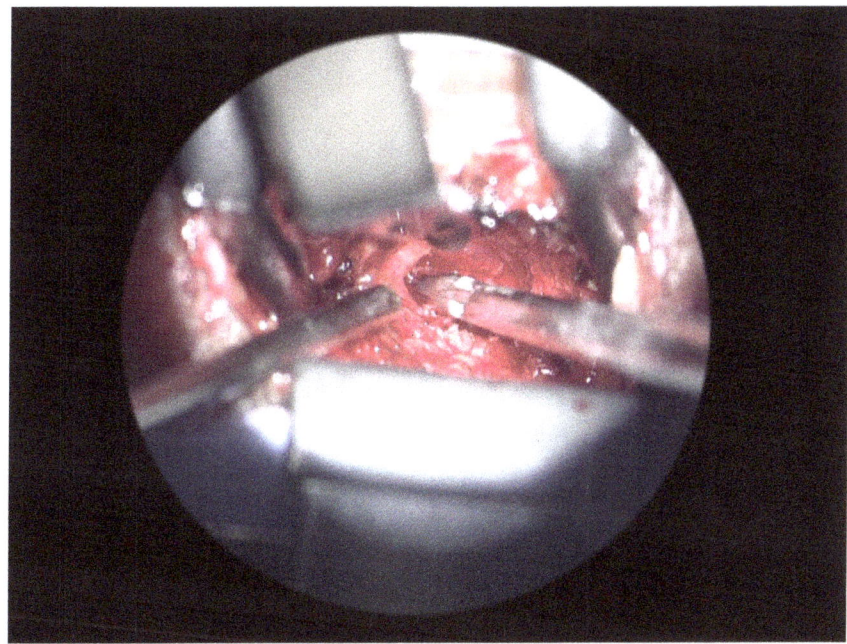

Fig. 3.143: Further exploration done to fish out hidden disc fragments

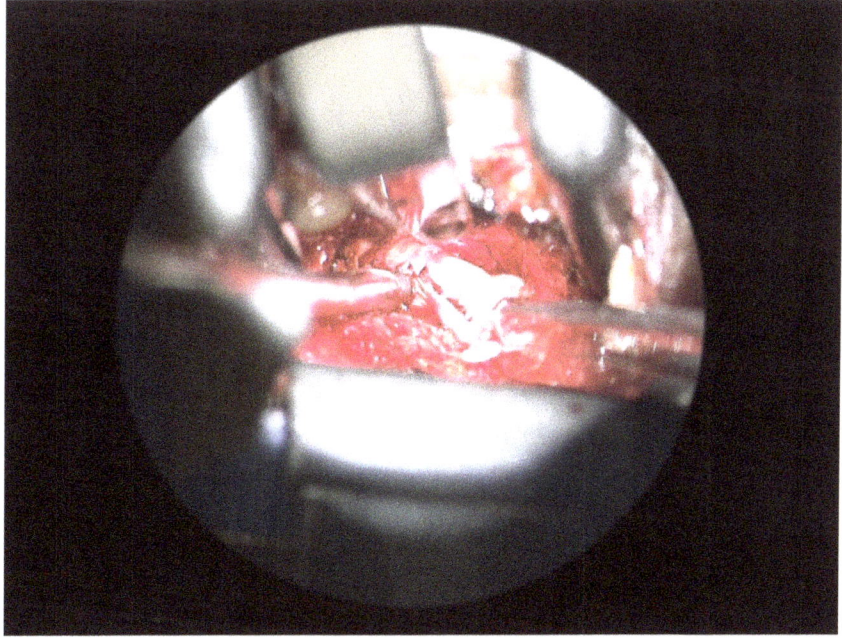

Fig. 3.144: Final fragments fished out

Superior Migration—Lateral

Case example: L_4/L_5 disc prolapse and superior migration of disc materials on the left side.

Clinical status: Middle-age man had severe left leg pain with classical sciatica and neurological deficit in the form of sensory deficit over L_5 dermatome and EHL weakness on left side. Many years ago, he had undergone laminectomy of L_5 and S_1 vertebrae for L_5/S_1 disc prolapse **(Figs 3.145 and 3.146)**.

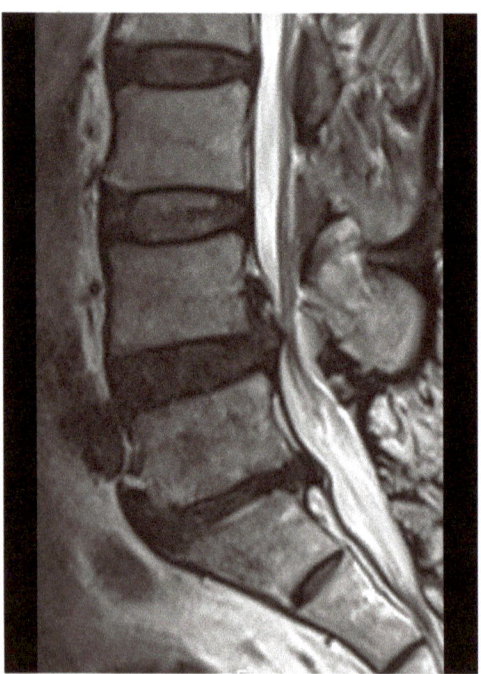

Fig. 3.145: MRI sagittal view showing L_4/L_5 disc prolapse and superior migration of degenerated disc material. Spinolaminectomy of L_5 during previous surgery is also noted

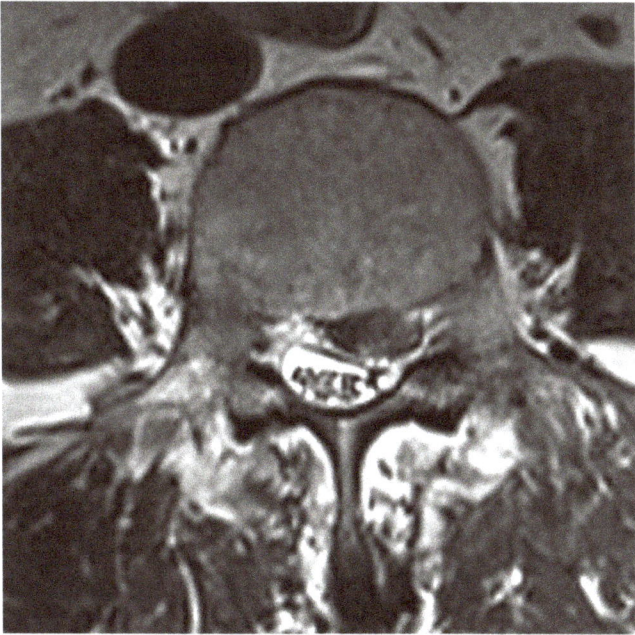

Fig. 3.146: MRI axial view showing disc material in the left lateral canal behind the posterior surface of vertebral body of L_4

Operative Procedure (Fig. 3.147A)

Step 1-Exposure of bony structures: Re-exploration is always challenging especially when the previous surgery was done many years ago. In this case, the L_5 spine and lamina was not present since laminectomy was done earlier. Through the previous midline incision over $L_4/L_5/S_1$, the paraspinal muscle dissected away from the midline through the scar tissue and the bony structures approached superiorly over L_4 spinous process and the facet joints laterally on left side **(Fig. 3.147B)**. I usually use a low cautery monopolar over the bones so that they are well delineated.

Step 2-Exposure of epidural space: The bony edges at facet joints and L_4 lamina identified. Medial half of facets drilled out **(Fig. 3.148)** and then the lamina of L_4 drilled out from its inferior margin **(Fig. 3.149)**. Later using appropriate Kerrisson punches lateral roof decompression and excison of three-fourths of L_4 lamina carried out **(Fig. 3.150)**. Epidural space below the bones is easier to dissect and the epidural fat and tissue can be appreciated. However, the tissues at the laminectomy site are tough and adherent to dura and nerve root sleeve. Care is taken to dissect them gently.

Neuro Spinal Surgery Operative Techniques: Micro Lumbar Discectomy

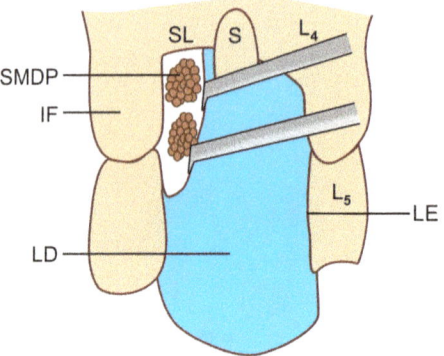

Fig. 3.147A
Abbreviations: SL, superior lamina; LE, laminectomy edge; IF, inferior facet; SMDP, superiorly migrated disc prolapse; LD, laminectomy dura

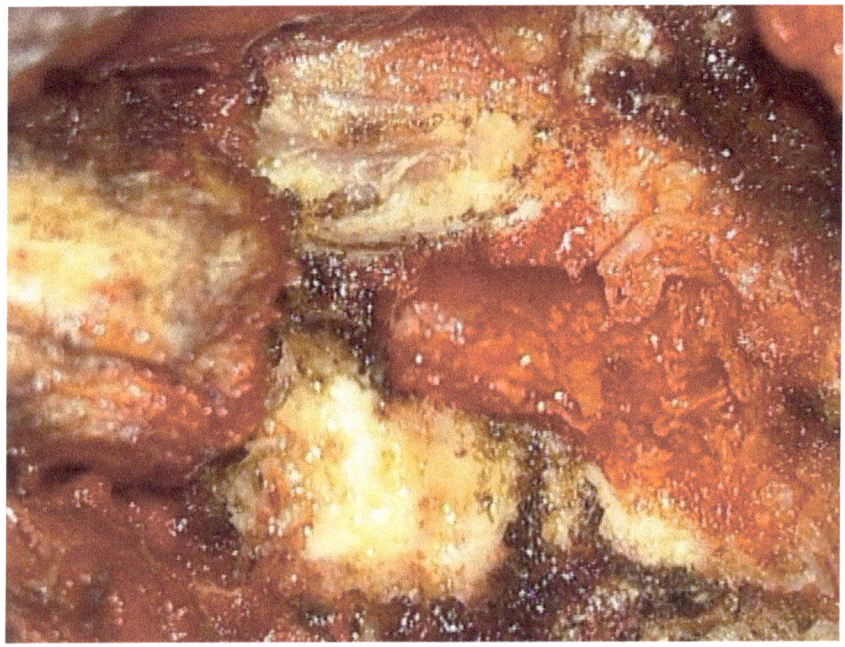

Fig. 3.147B: Re-exploration. L_4 spinous process and L_4/L_5 facet joint exposed. Note the large laminectomy defect

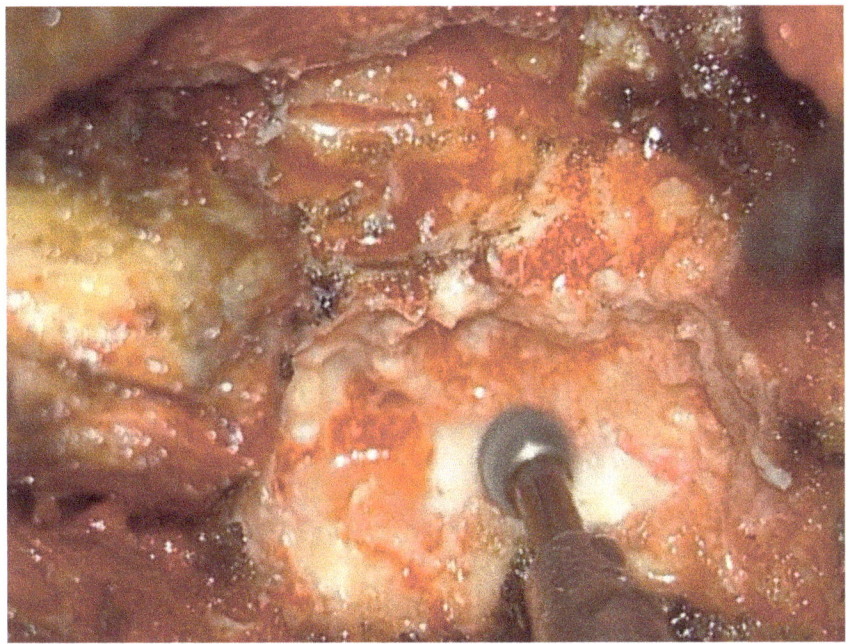

Fig. 3.148: Drilling of medial of facet joint

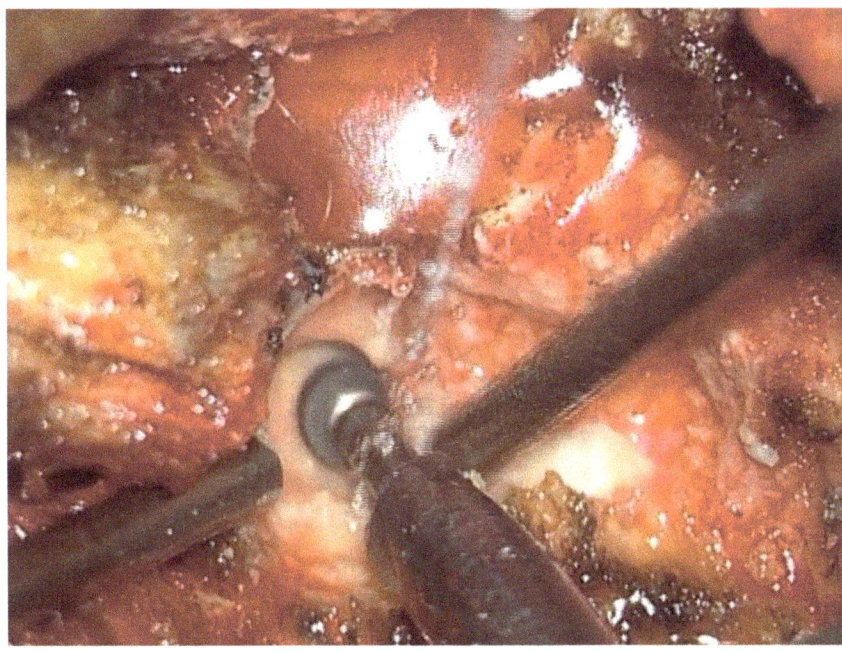

Fig. 3.149: Lower border of L_4 lamina drilling

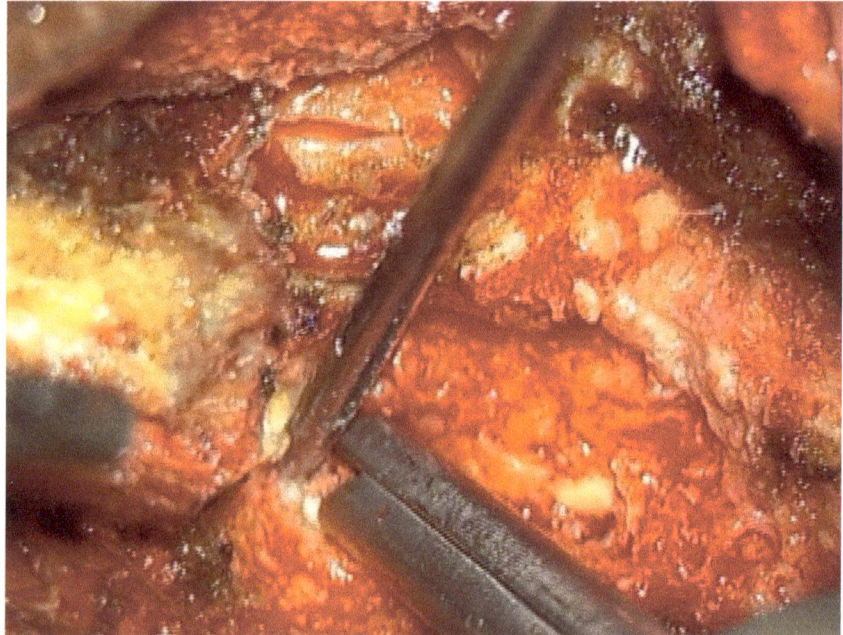

Fig. 3.150: Thinned out bones excised with Kerrison punch

Step 3-Discectomy and neural decompression: The shoulder region of L_5 nerve root retracted medially to expose the bulging L_4/L_5 disc initially **(Fig. 3.151)** and later the dura superiorly retracted by moving the retractor up until the superiorly migrated disc material reached **(Fig. 3.152)**. The superiorly migrated materials actually were placed in the lateral canal behind the posterior wall of the vertebral body and the same hooked out and removed with disc punches **(Fig. 3.153)**. Thorough search for migrated disc materials carried out and search followed to disc level. Bulging annulus cut and remaining degenerated disc materials removed until satisfactory neural decompression was achieved **(Fig. 3.154)**.

Operative Techniques with Case Examples | 103

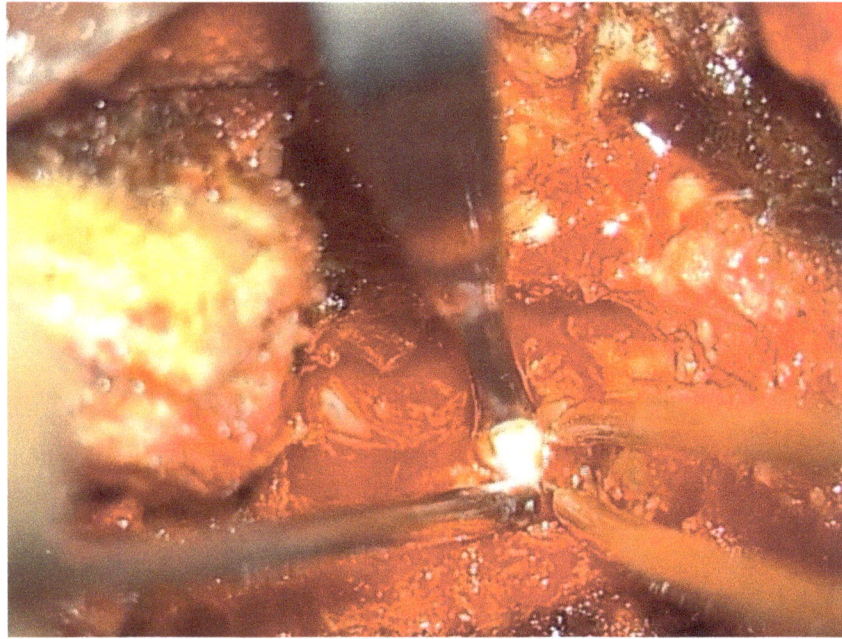

Fig. 3.151: Nerve root retracted medially over the bulging disc

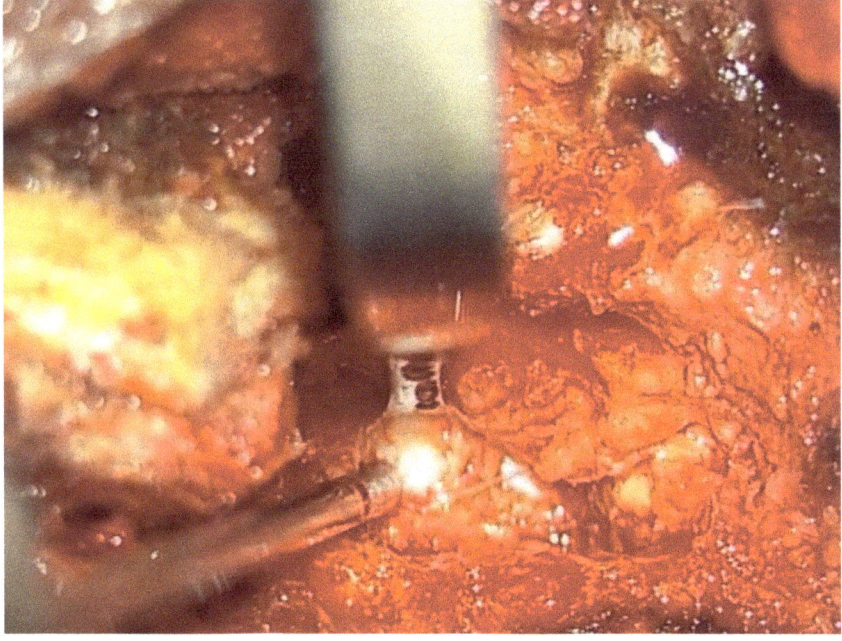

Fig. 3.152: Subsequently, the nerve root retracted superiorly to expose superiorly migrated fragments

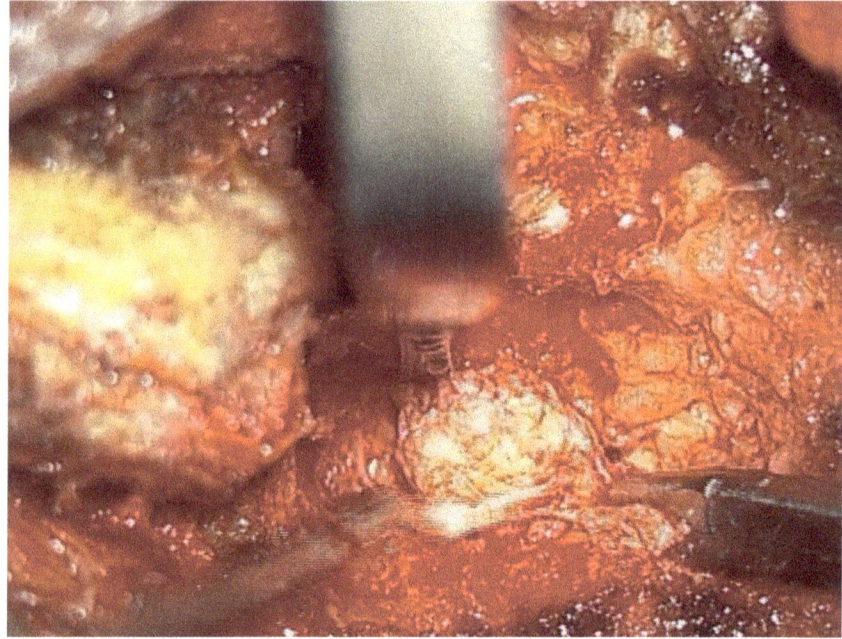

Fig. 3.153: The fragments are removed with disc punches

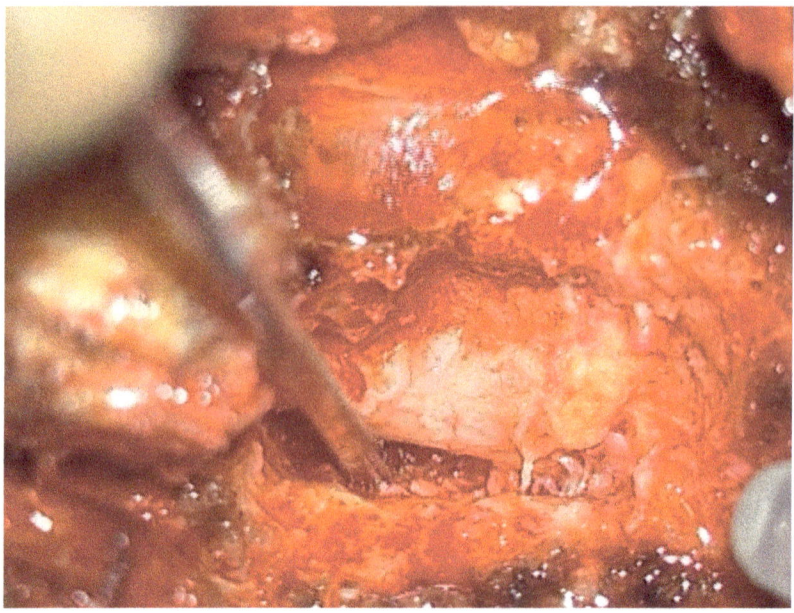

Fig. 3.154: Dura and nerve root free completely in lateral canal

RECURRENT DISC PROLAPSE

Recurrent Disc Prolapse (Acute and Small)

Case example: L_4/L_5 recurrent disc prolapse and inferior migration of the disc material in the foramen on the left side.

Clinical status: A middle-aged lady who underwent micro lumbar discectomy one week ago presented to us with aggravating pain on the same leg with higher intensity following squatting in the postoperative period. Earlier she had complete pain relief following micro lumbar discectomy for L_4/L_5 disc prolapse. A large firm degenerated disc material was excised from the lateral canal and the nerve root was confirmed lax. Intradiscal fragments were also removed. Latest MRI showed recurrent disc prolapse on the same side (left) at L_4/L_5 level and the fragments migrating inferiorly in lateral canal **(Figs 3.155 to 3.158)**.

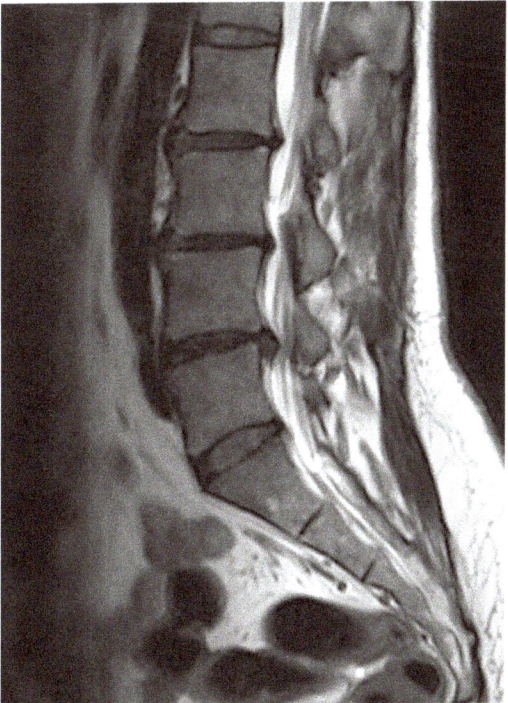

Fig. 3.155: MRI sagittal view showing L_4/L_5 disc prolapse before first surgery

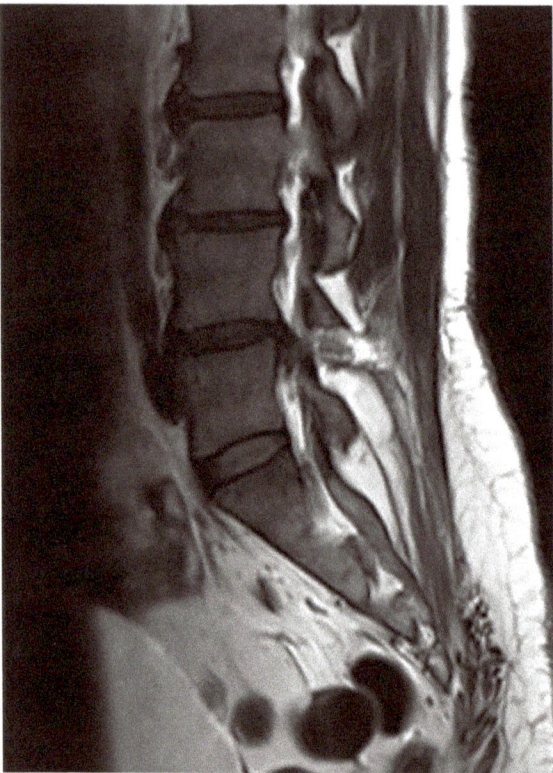

Fig. 3.156: MRI sagittal view showing recurrent disc prolapse

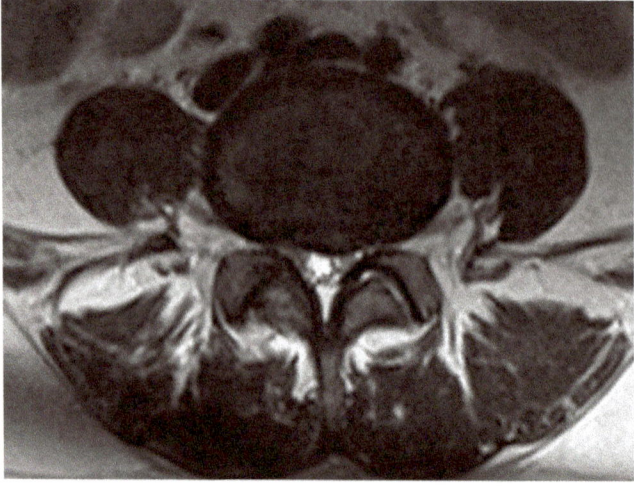

Fig. 3.157: MRI axial view showing L_4/L_5 disc prolapse before first surgery

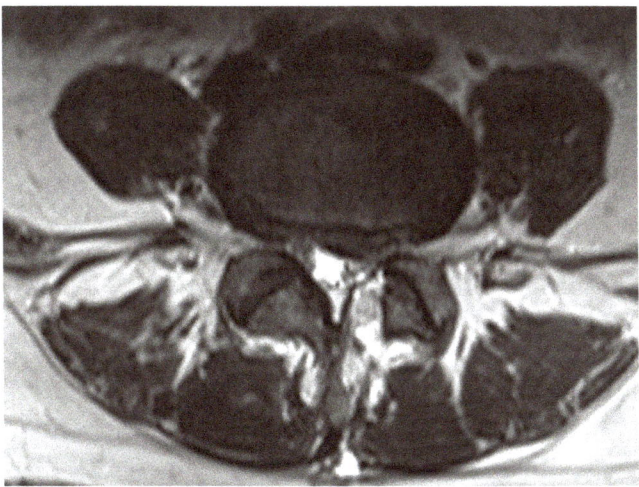

Fig. 3.158: MRI axial view showing recurrent disc prolapse

Operative Procedure

Step 1-Exposure of the interlaminar space: Revision surgery is always a challenge and the tissue planes are not clear due fibrosis and adhesions. The skin was incised and paraspinal muscles were dissected away from the bone using low current monoploar. Dissection was carried always over the bone surface and the laminotomy defect created earlier during the previous surgery was demarcated well. Subsequently, using 15 blade knife, the fibrous tissue was cut in the interlaminar space. Here surgeon should take precaution not to venture deep with the knife. Tissue forceps were used along with blunt hooks until the epidural space was exposed. Lack of ligamentum flavum was challenging since dura and nerve root were exposed with fibrous tissue over them. However, hemostats used in first surgery were of help in exposure of the space above and nerve root below as seen in this case **(Fig. 3.159)**.

Step 2-Exposure of dura, nerve root and disc: Using blunt hooks and rasperators, the soft tissues such as the organized hemostats removed **(Fig. 3.160)** and gentle dissection continued from lateral to medial to delineate the nerve root. Fibrous strands and tissues dissected meticulously in places where the ligamentum was not excised the adhesions were more around dura **(Fig. 3.161)**. We never used force to pull out adhesive bands from dura and nerve root sleeves. Usually dura over roots are not shiny and hence need to be careful while retracting the root medially. A firm dissection over the disc area with a blunt edge instrument like rasperator can be of much help in these situations **(Fig. 3.162)**. No bony removal was done since the disc prolapse was seen medial to the already trimmed out facets during the previous surgery.

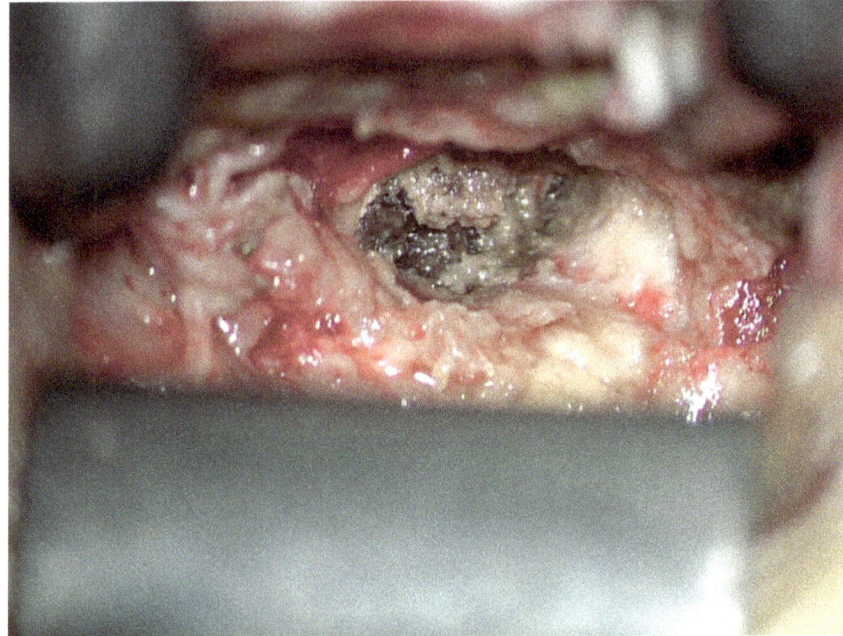

Fig. 3.159: Interlaminar space opened and note the organized hemostats

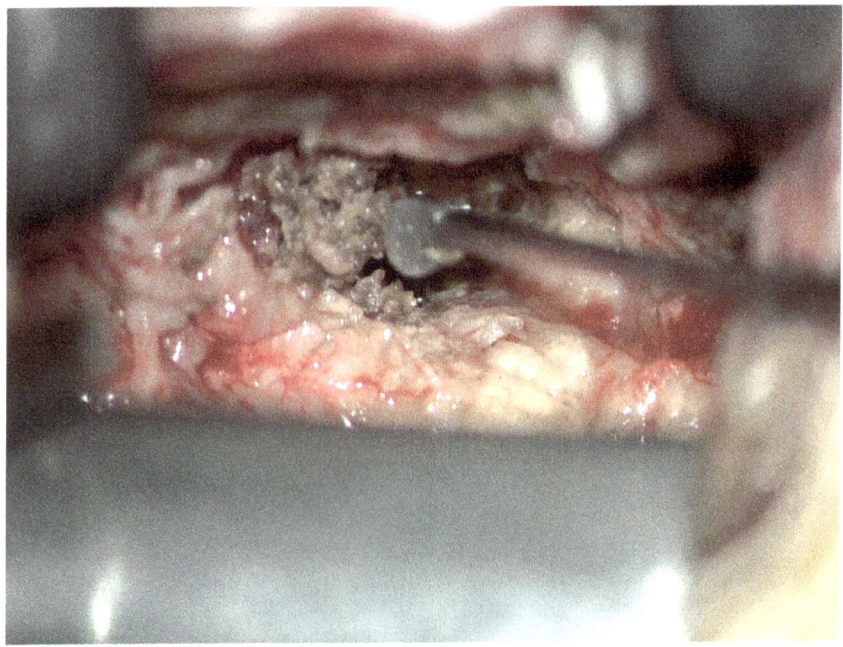

Fig. 3.160: Hemostats are removed

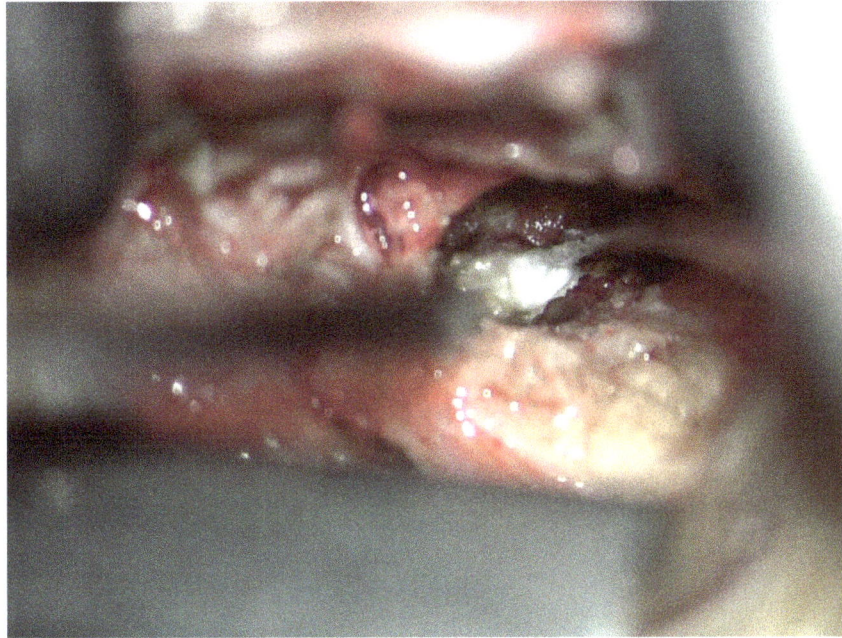

Fig. 3.161: Nerve root is visualized and it is not shiny as in fresh cases. Lateral to it is seen white disc material

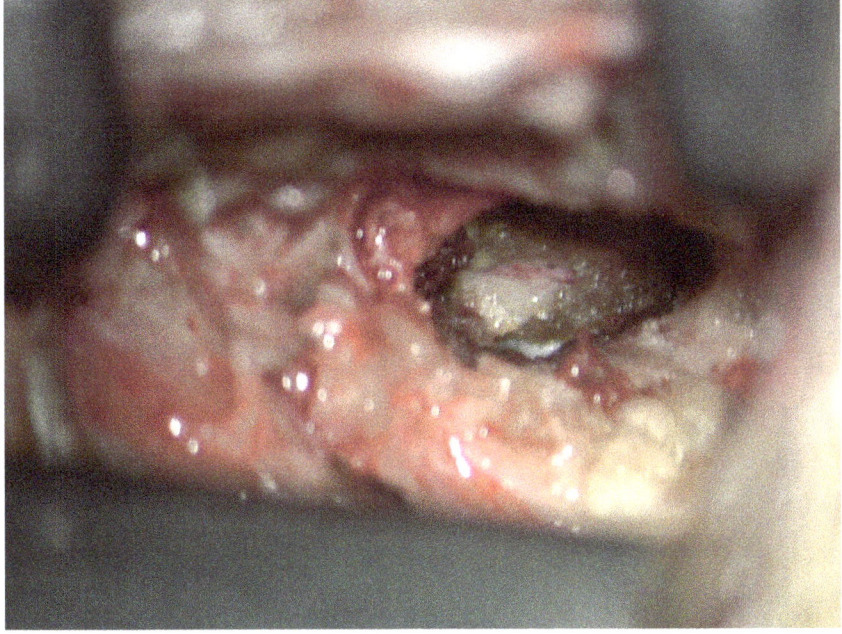

Fig. 3.162: Nerve root retracted medially to expose disc material

Step 3–Discectomy and nerve root decompression: Nerve root seen stretched by underlying disc retracted and soft white disc fragments removed **(Fig. 3.163)**. Nerve root was retracted further down to expose inferiorly migrated fragments **(Fig. 3.164)**. The same were removed and intradiscal fishing out was done aggressively to prevent another recurrence **(Fig. 3.165)**. Disc space and the upper posterior wall of the lower vertebra seen clearly thus confirming removal of entire recurrent disc prolapse **(Fig. 3.166)**. The nerve root seen free and pulsatile and the root canal found extremely free **(Fig. 3.167)**.

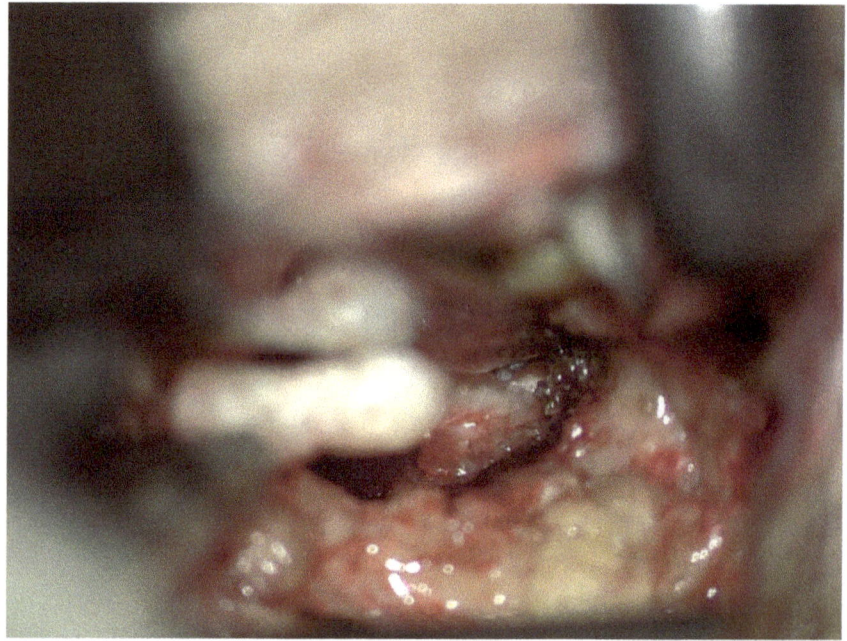

Fig. 3.163: Fragment removed

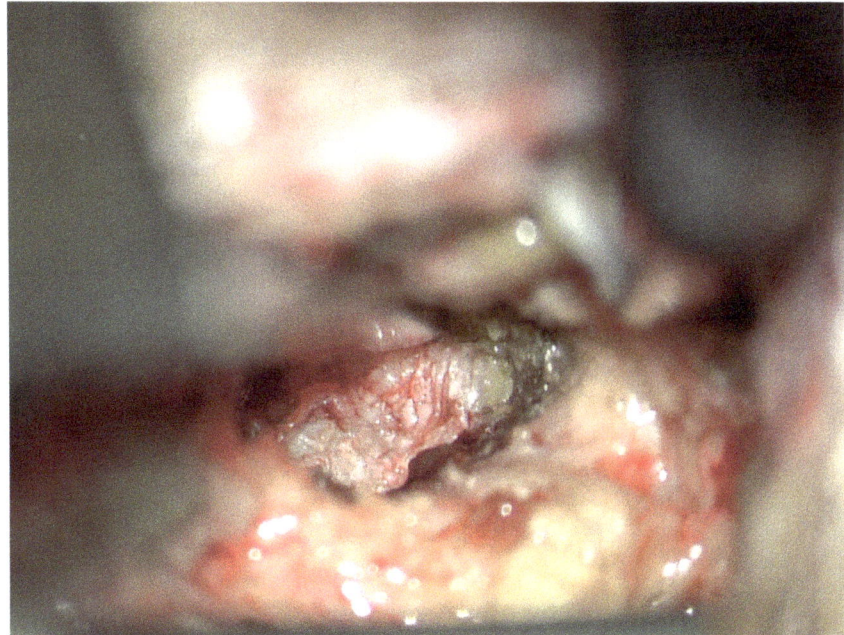

Fig. 3.164: Further exploration brings out more fragments and they are removed as well

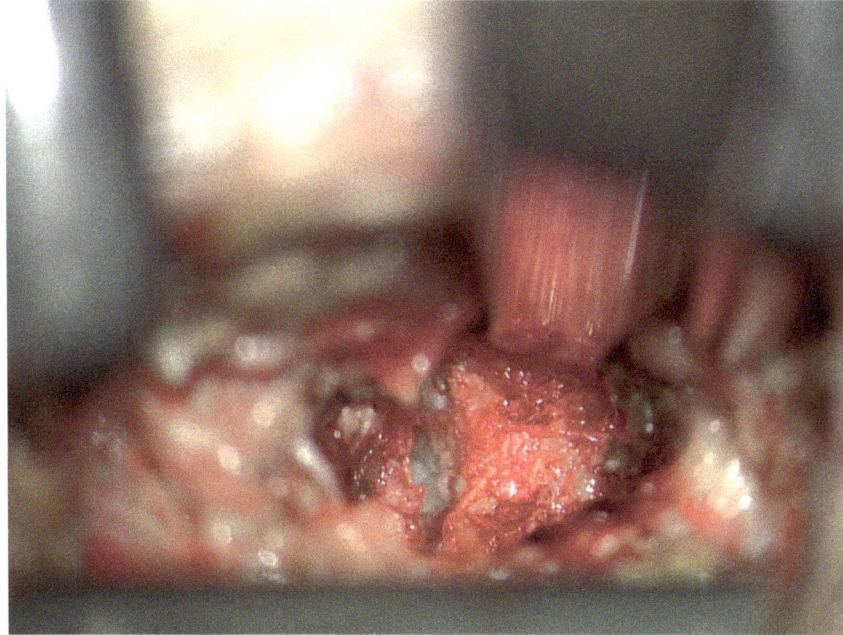

Fig. 3.165: Nerve root still retracted medially and the disc space explored further

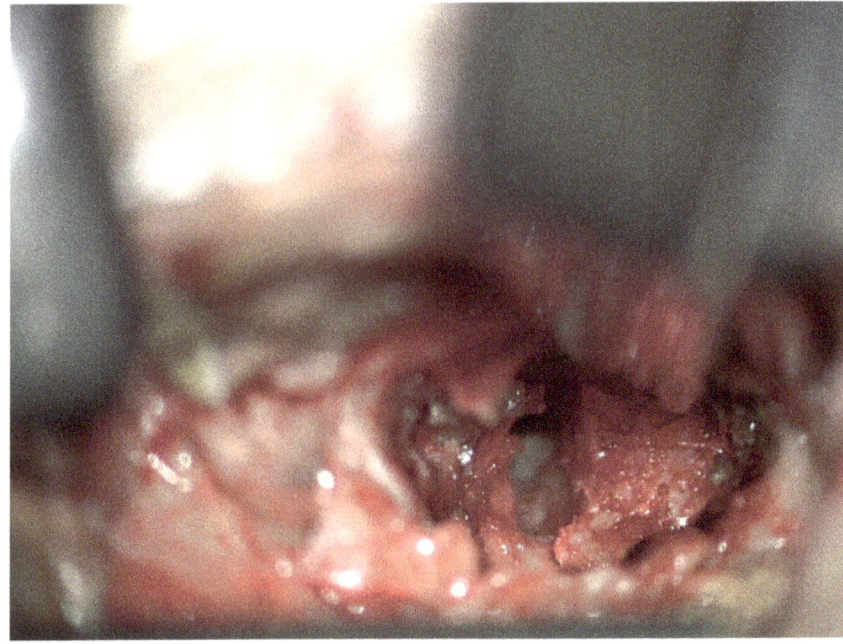

Fig. 3.166: Note the intradiscal space and the free epidural space

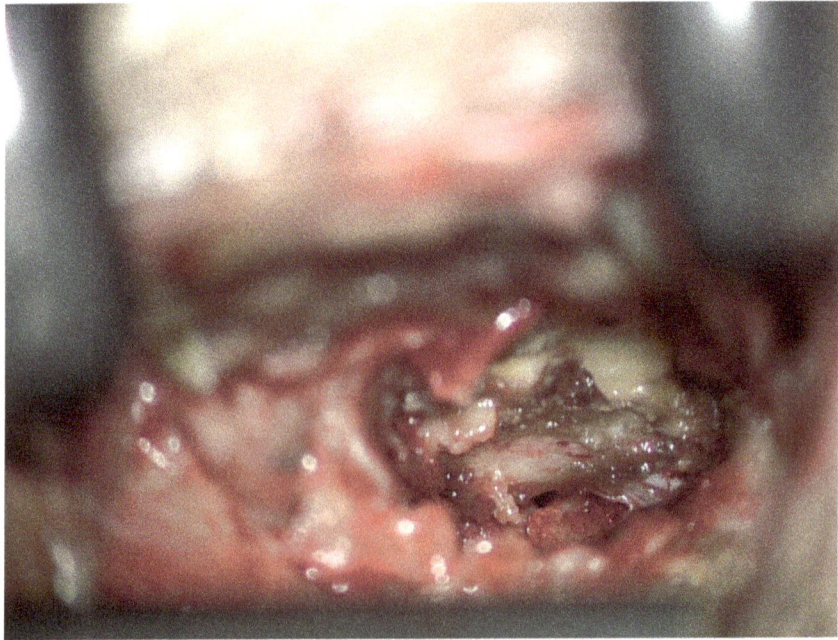

Fig. 3.167: Relaxed nerve root after complete removal of recurrent disc fragments

Recurrent Disc Prolapse (Chronic and Large)

Case example: L_4/L_5 recurrent disc prolapse centrolateral.

Clinical status: Middle-age lady presented with left sciatica of six months duration. The pain was intermittent and was thought to be cyclical with menstrual periods. The patient had undergone micro lumbar discectomy 2 years ago for left sciatica and was asymptomatic for eighteen months **(Figs 3.168 to 3.171)**.

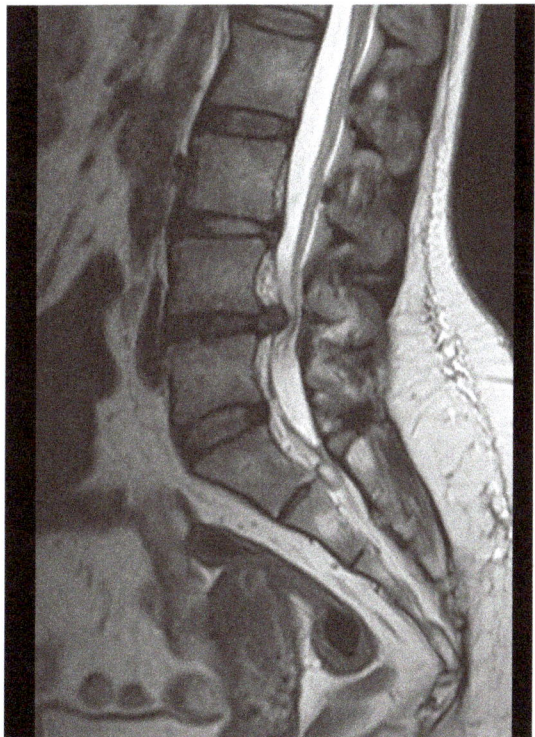

Fig. 3.168: MRI sagittal view showing a large disc prolapse at L_4/L_5 level before first surgery

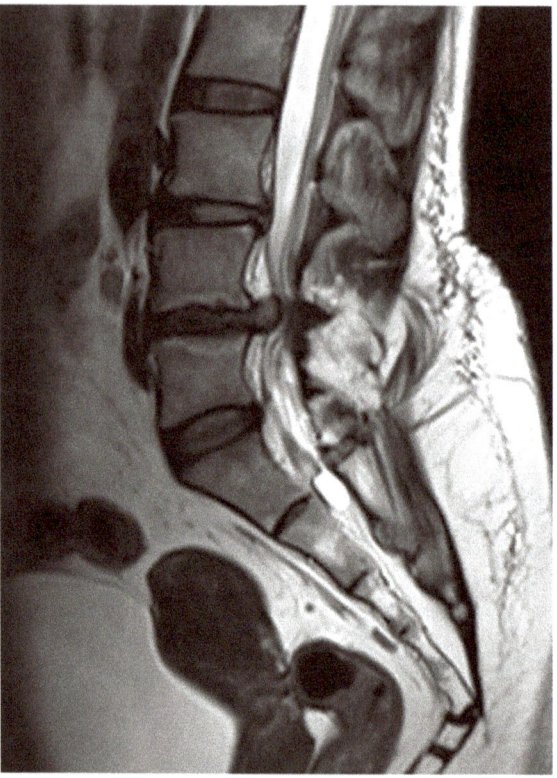

Fig. 3.169: MRI sagittal view showing recurrent disc prolapse after eighteen months

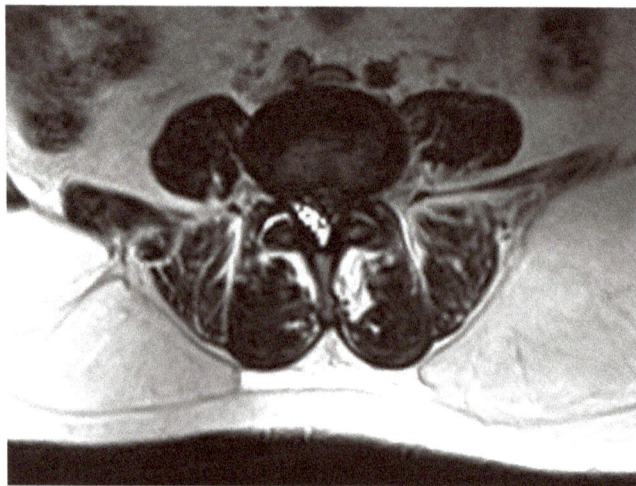

Fig. 3.170: MRI axial view showing lateral disc prolapse before first surgery

Operative Techniques with Case Examples | 115

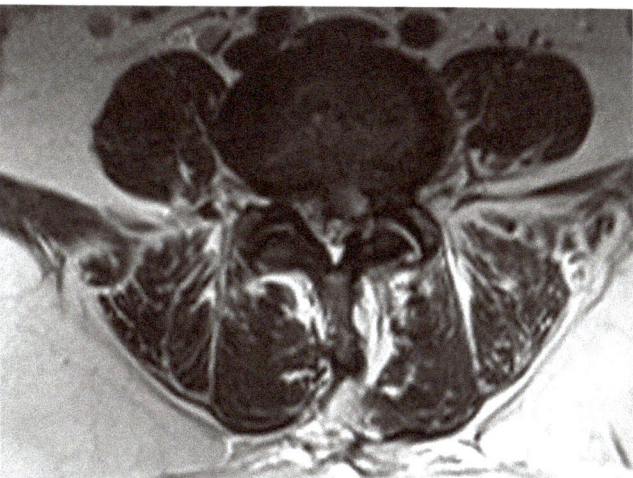

Fig. 3.171: MRI axial view showing recurrent disc prolapse lateral and foraminal after eighteen months

Operative Procedure

Step 1–Exposure of the shoulder side of nerve root: In this case, the interlaminar area was exposed as in the previous case. Here the superior lamina and the facets, interlaminar space along with adherent ligamentum flavum were exposed well **(Fig. 3.172)**. The superior lamina and medial surface of inferior facet of the superior vertebra drilled out until the inner table was reached **(Figs 3.173 and 3.174)**. Then using the Kerrison punch, the bone excised to expose the epidural space that was not violated during the previous surgery **(Fig. 3.175)**. This is the key point. Exploration should start from a site where normal anatomy could be appreciated. This step makes the surgeon easy in identifying the structures and avoid neurological deficit and dural tear. The nerve root was seen covered by a dull dura and less shiny as in fresh cases **(Fig. 3.176)**. In some places, it was difficult to dissect the dura away from the recurrent disc underneath. The shoulder of the nerve root was demarcated and using a rasperator the nerve root retracted to expose the entire recurrent disc material in the epidural space **(Fig. 3.177)**.

Step 2–Discectomy and lateral canal deroofing: The extruded recurrent disc materials were removed **(Fig. 3.178)**. In this case, they were more fibrous and firmer **(Fig. 3.179)**. The intradiscal region was searched thoroughly for free materials and fished out. The nerve root was seen lax but still had fibrous tissue inferiorly. Further removal of medial aspect of facet of inferior vertebra was fashioned by Kerrison punch and the entire lateral canal was decompressed **(Fig. 3.180)**.

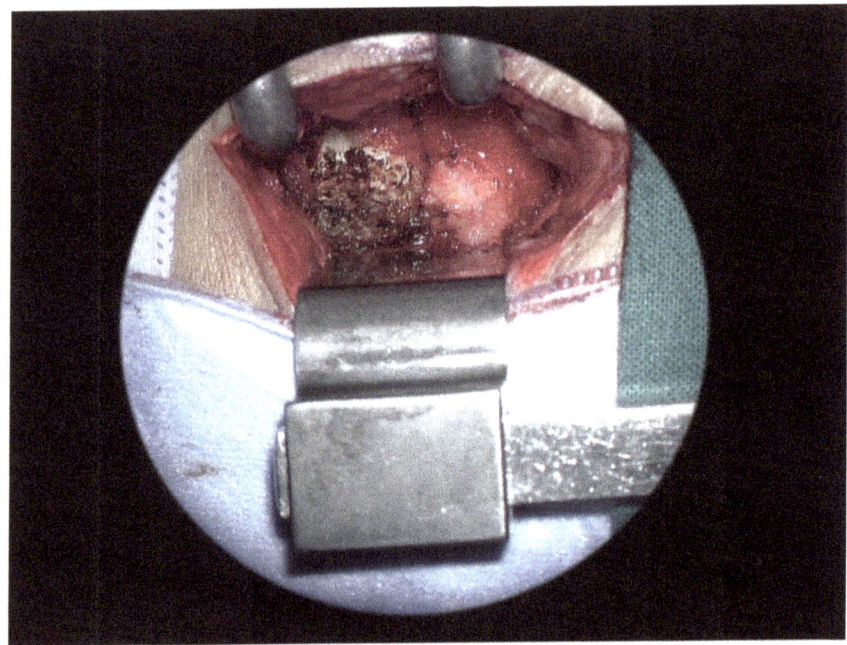

Fig. 3.172: Intrelaminar space exposed

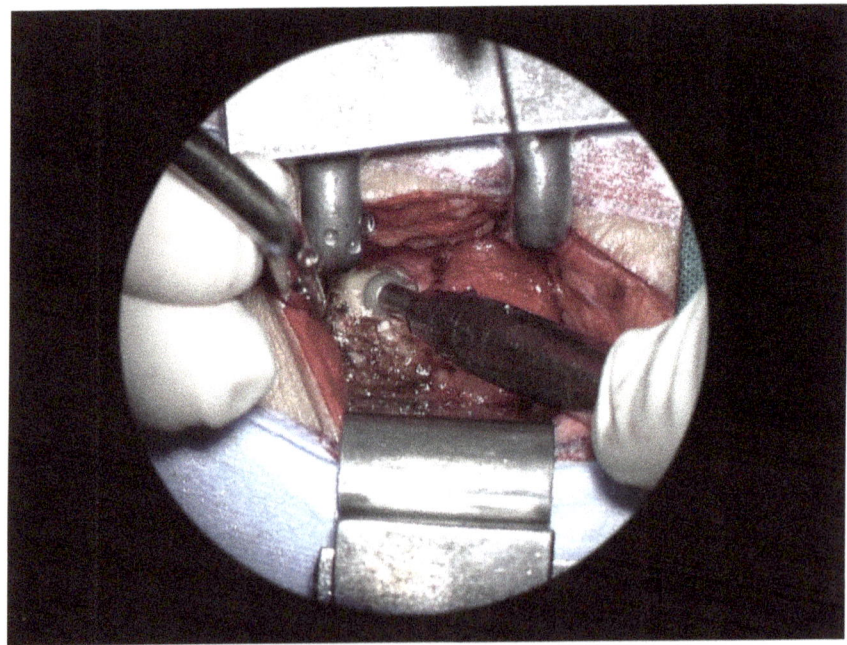

Fig. 3.173: Upper lamina drilled out

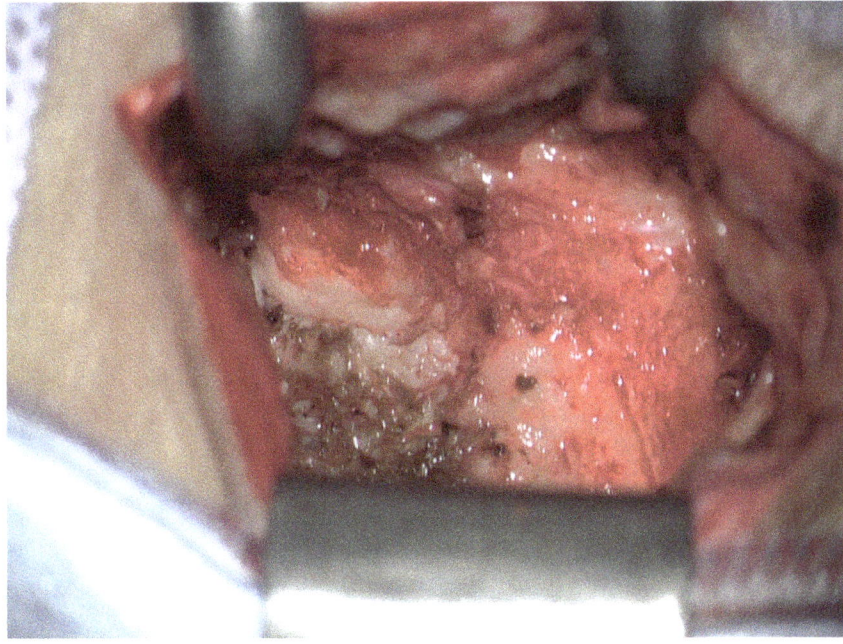

Fig. 3.174: Medial facetectomy and inferior edge of upper lamina drilled

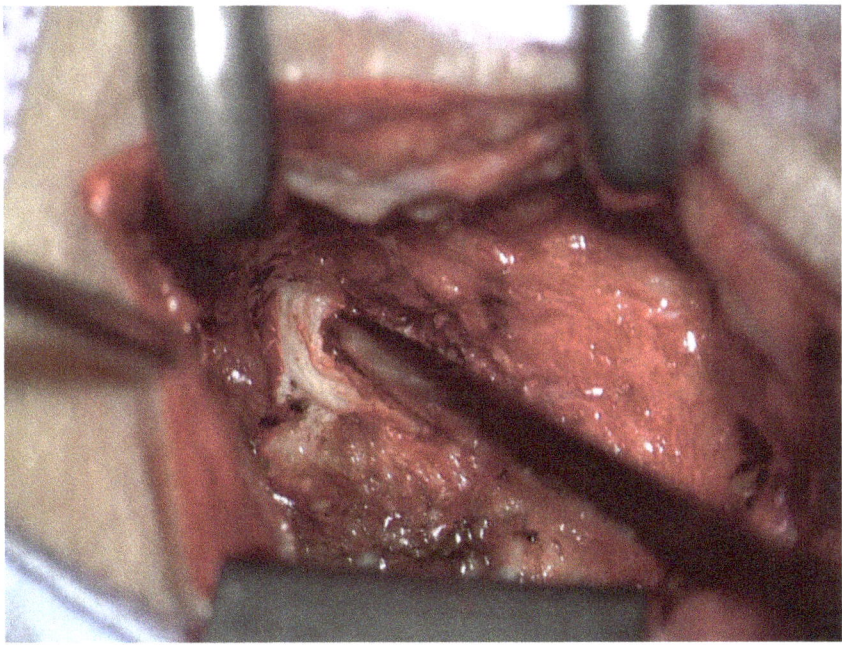

Fig. 3.175: Using Kerrison punch thinned out bones excised

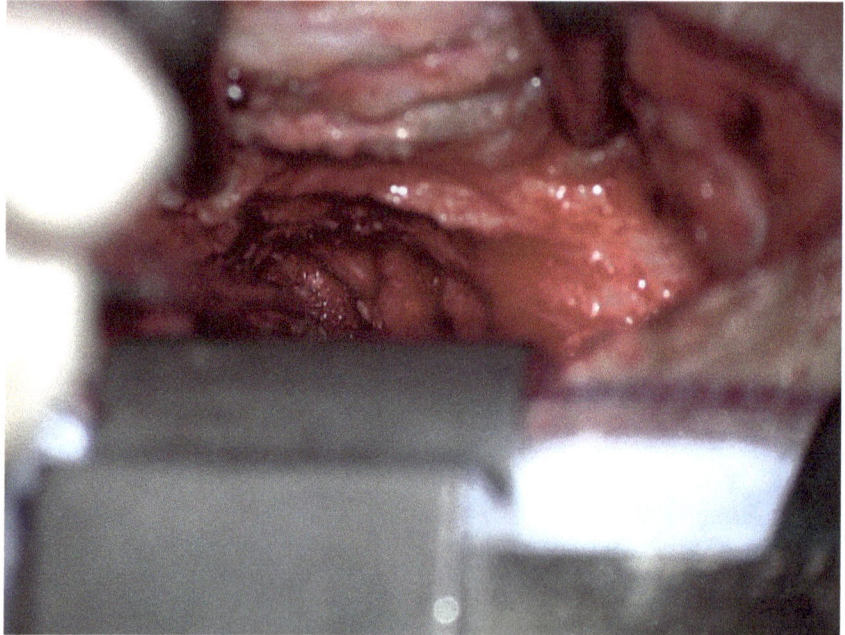

Fig. 3.176: Nerve root is exposed and note the dull texture of nerve root

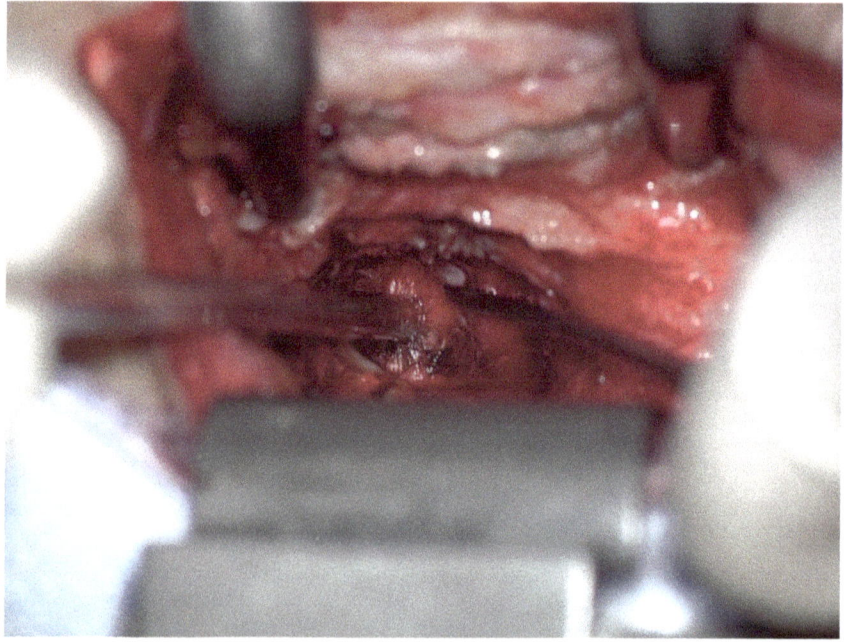

Fig. 3.177: Nerve root retracted and bulging annulus exposed

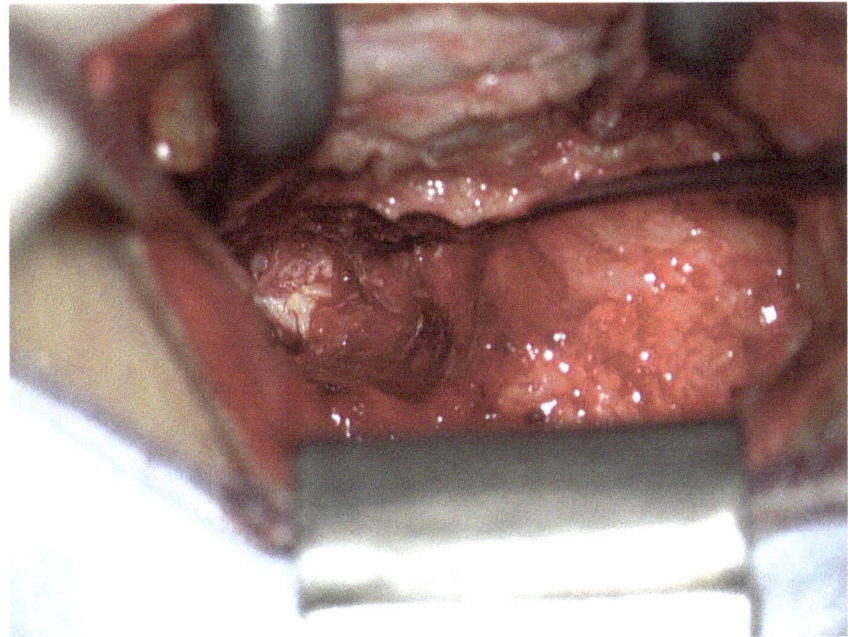

Fig. 3.178: Sub-annular degenerated disc fragment

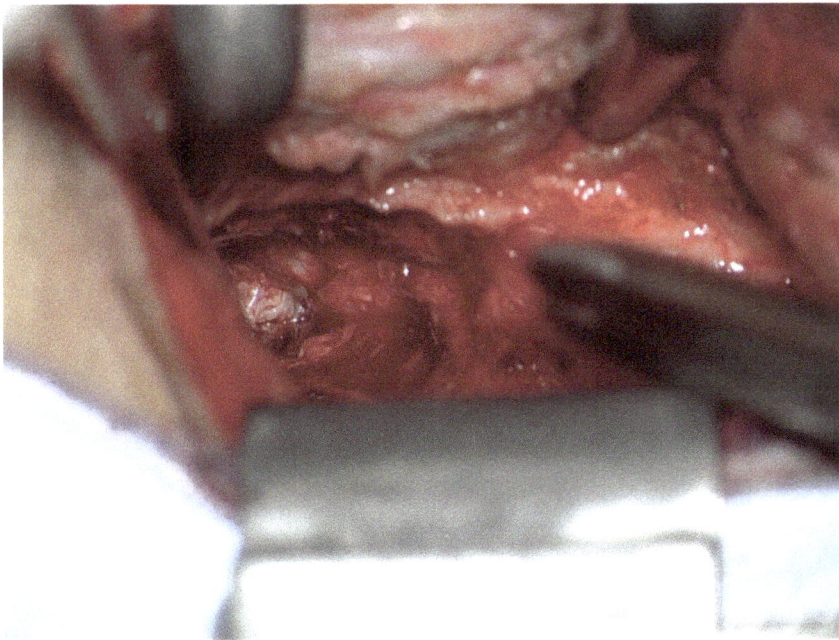

Fig. 3.179: Fragments are fibrous and hard and removed

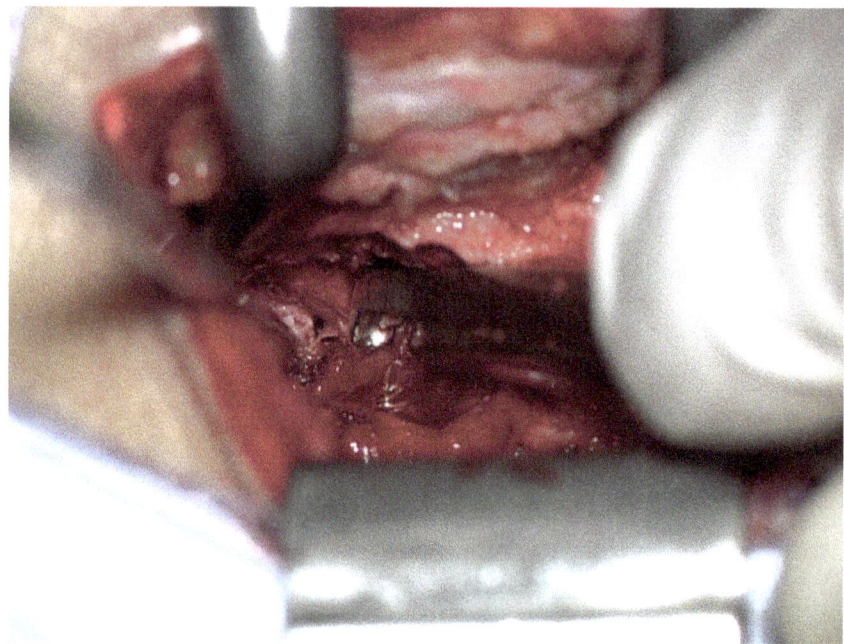

Fig. 3.180: Now lateral canal deroofing performed

Step 3-Excision of epidural fibrosis: Though, in this case, the recurrent disc was the cause of symptoms and was the indication for surgery, significant fibrous tissue was seen over inferior half of the nerve root **(Fig. 3.181)**. In such situations, care must be taken not to damage the dura over the entire nerve root. Sharp hooks were used along with microscissors to gently peel out the strands over the nerve root and excised without traction **(Fig. 3.182)**. The technique of peeling of these tissues were along the nerve root and never was across. If the tissues are very adherent I usually leave them as in this case since the recurrent disc was obviously the cause and it was not an isolated perineural fibrosis. Hemostasis was secured and a good irrigation of saline with steroids was done at the end **(Fig. 3.183)**.

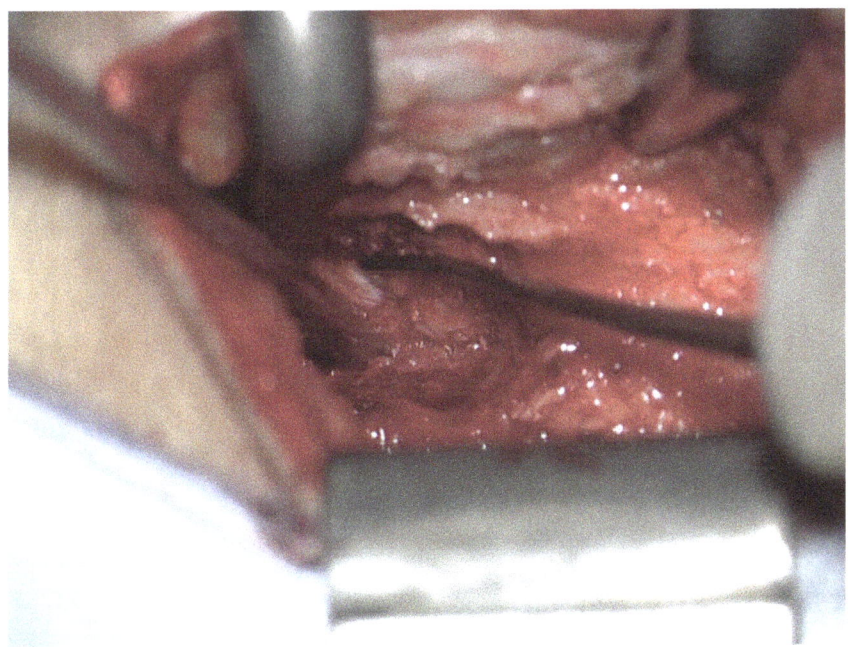

Fig. 3.181: Nerve root is seen better above than inferiorly. Adherent tissues over nerve sheath

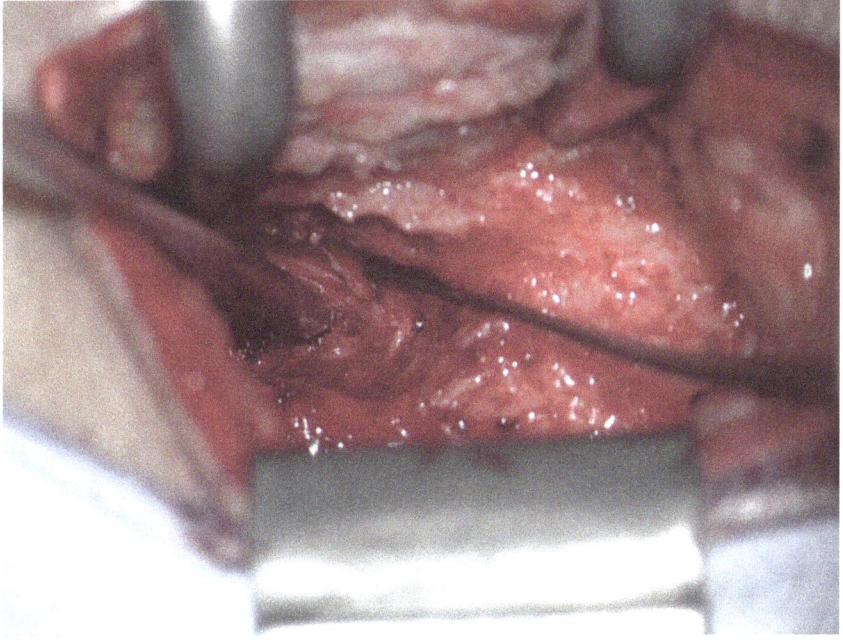

Fig. 3.182: Fibrous tissues dissected from dural sleeve without creating a rent

Neuro Spinal Surgery Operative Techniques: Micro Lumbar Discectomy

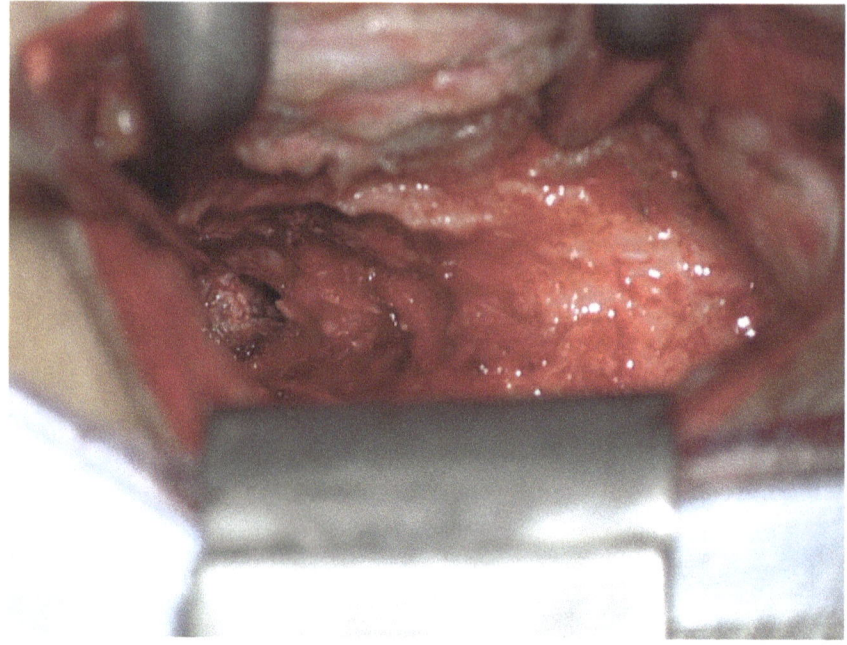

Fig. 3.183: Entire nerve root freed at the end

Far-lateral Disc Prolapse (Shoulder Approach)

Case Example 1

A case far-lateral disc prolapse on the right side compressing the exiting nerve root (L_3) at the level of L_3/L_4 disc level **(Fig. 3.184)**.

Clinical status: Young man with severe pain over the anterior aspect of right thigh associated with sensory deficit and absent knee jerk.

Operative Procedure (Fig. 3.185A)

Foraminotomy and Discectomy (Shoulder Approach)

Step 1–Level marking: Far-lateral disc prolapses are approached through the neural foramen from the lateral side and the foramen is in line with the base of spinous process in lateral view. Hence after positioning, the patient as we do, for all MLD patients, the level is marked with a needle placed on the side of spinous process that corresponds to the foramen of interest. For example, in this case of L_3/L_4 the base of L_3 spinous process is marked and the skin incision marked just lateral to the spinous process **(Figs 3.185B and C)**.

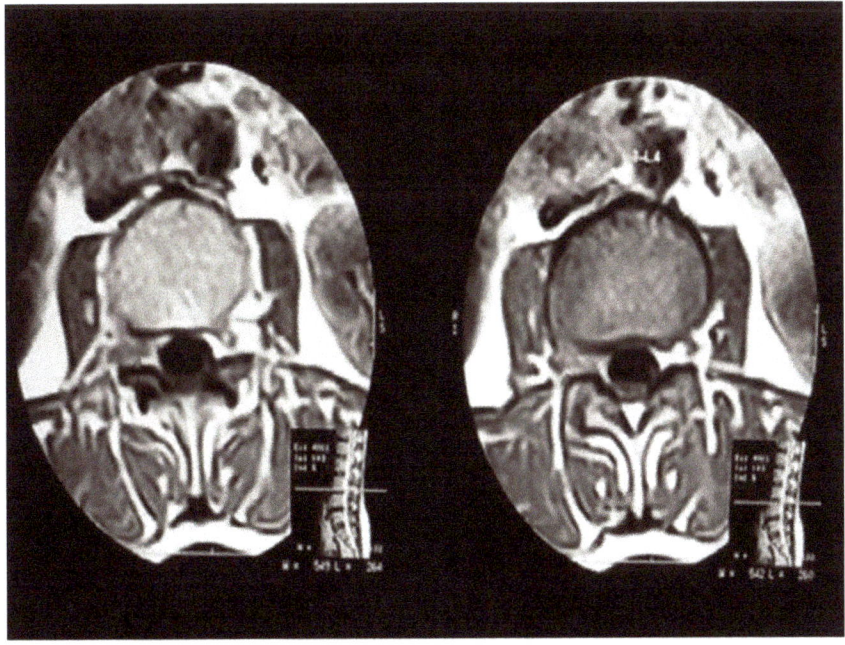

Fig. 3.184: MRI axial cut showing far lateral disc prolapse

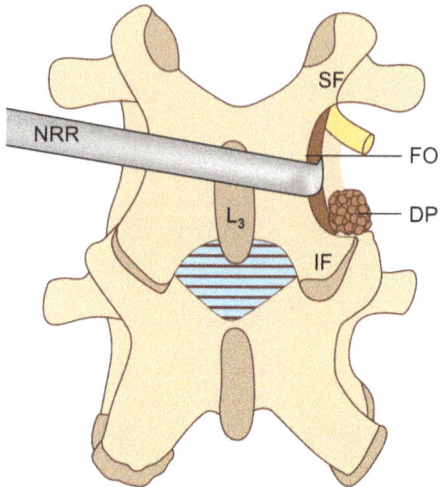

Fig. 3.185A Foraminotomy
Abbreviations: DP, disc prolapse; FO, foraminotomy edge of pars; IF, inferior facet; NRR, nerve root retractor; SF, superior facet

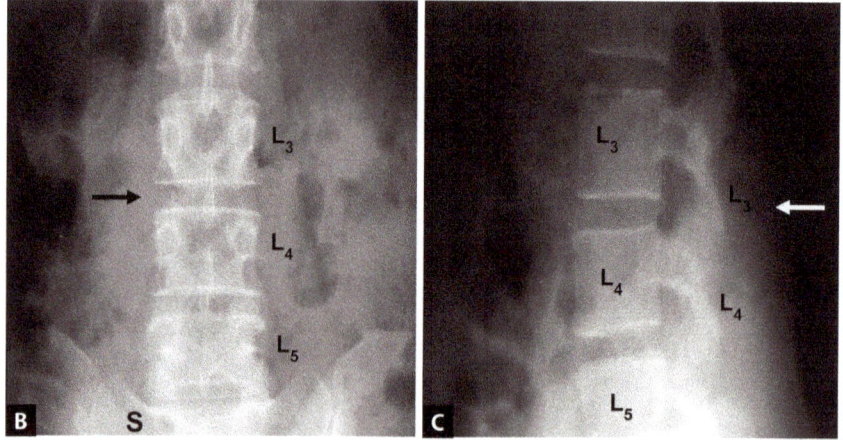

Figs 3.185B and C: (B) X-ray masking: AP view; (C) X-ray masking: Lateral view

Step 2-Exposure of foramen: The paraspinal muscle is retracted from L_3 spinous process along the lamina on the right side until lateral edge of pars is visualized **(Figs 3.186A and B)**. Dissection is carried out to expose the L_3/L_4 facet joint capsule below and the inferior edge of L_2 facet above and the area lateral to the pars. Pars inter-articularis has a smooth curve on the lateral aspect and is the bridge between superior and inferior facets **(Fig. 3.187A)**. Lateral edge of pars is drilled out **(Fig. 3.187B)** and the bones excised with Kerrison punches **(Fig. 3.187C)**. Sometimes, the lateral edge of inferior facet is also drilled out depending on the position of prolapsed disc material.

Operative Techniques with Case Examples

This procedure opens the foramen from posterior and allows access to far lateral, foraminal and axillary disc materials.

Step 3–Discectomy: The ligamentum flavum thus exposed is now removed **(Fig. 3.187D)** and careful dissection of foraminal region will expose the prolapsed disc material, which can be removed meticulously **(Figs 3.187E to G)**. The nerve root that traverses out below the pars can be visualized after discectomy. The nerve root traversing down can be retracted to explore more medially.

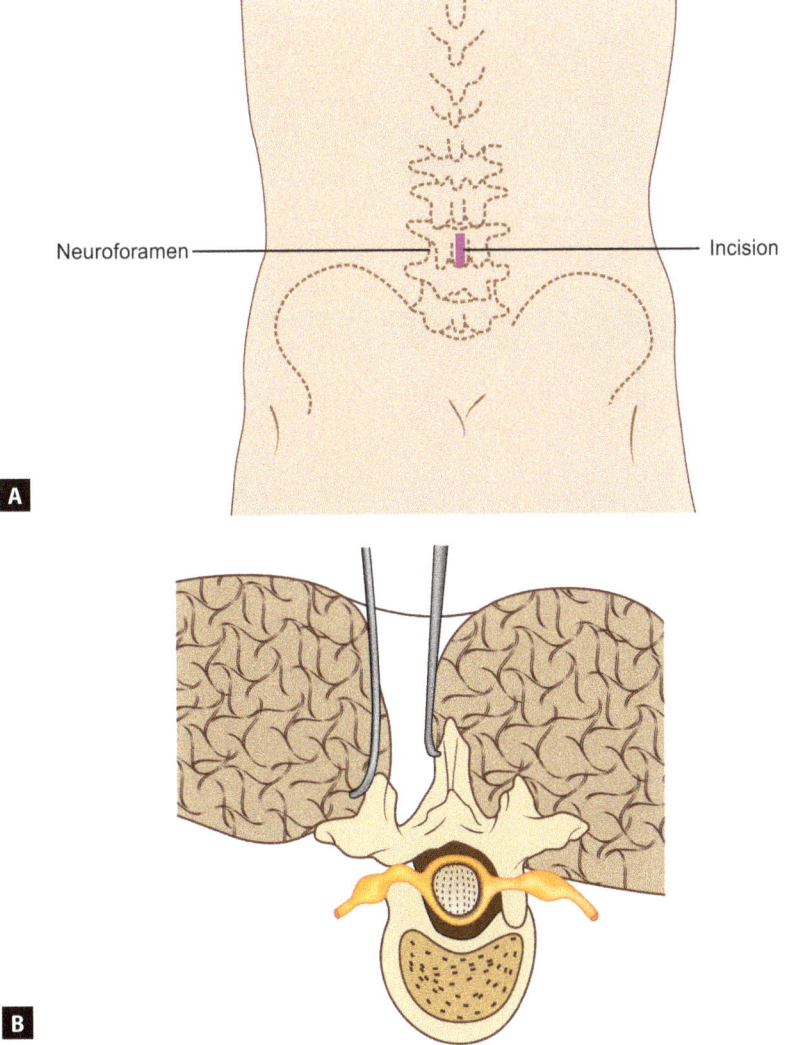

Figs 3.186A and B: (A) Incision over the spinous process that corresponds to the level; (B) Paraspinal retraction as done in MLD but up to lateral edge of pars

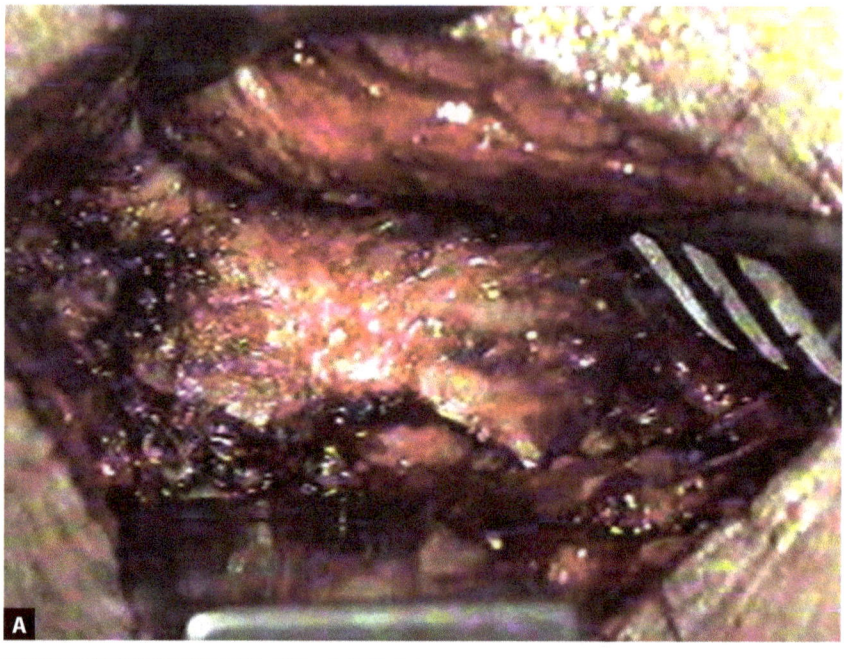
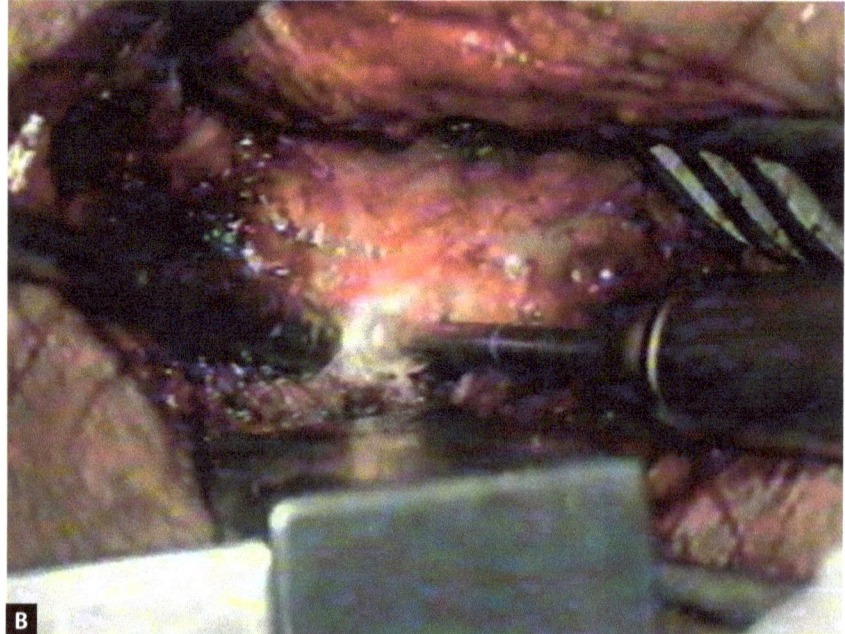

Figs 3.187A and B

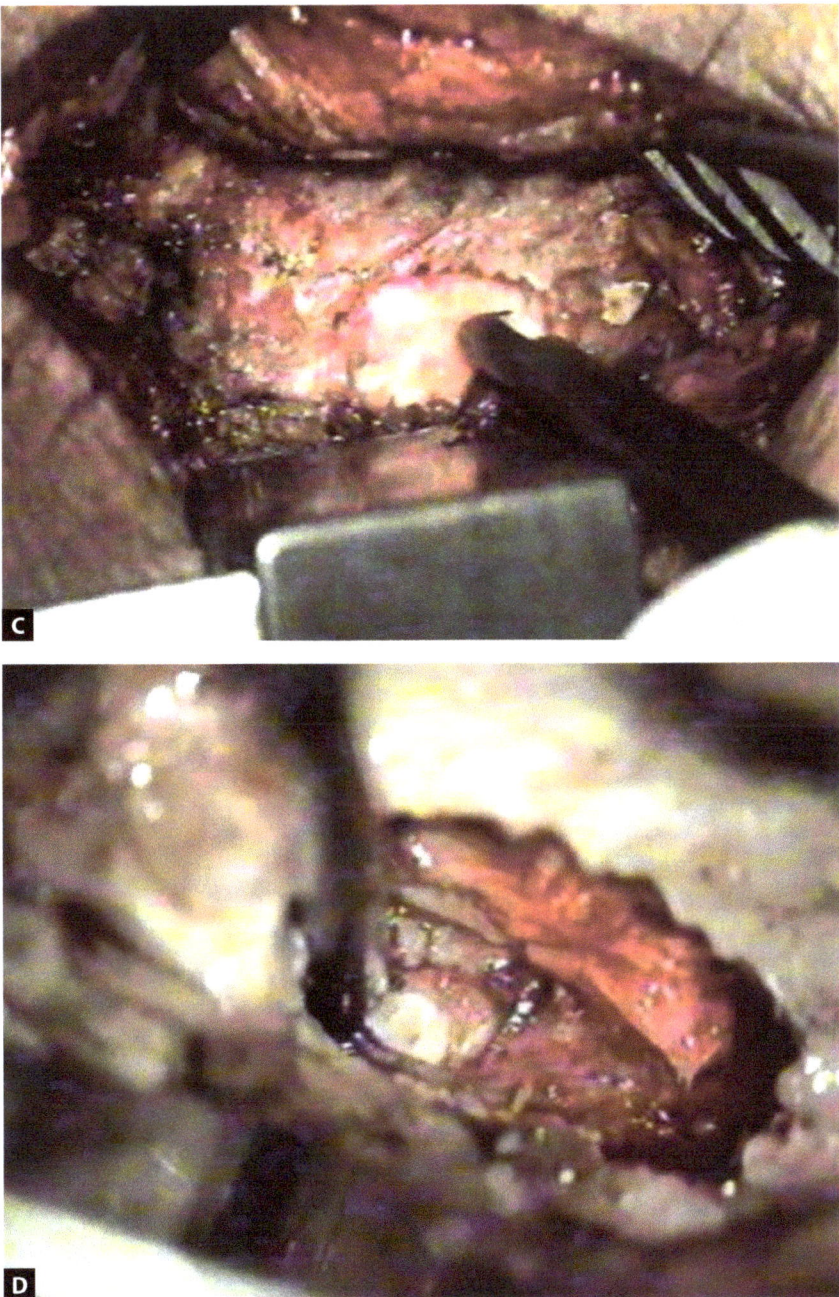

Figs 3.187C and D

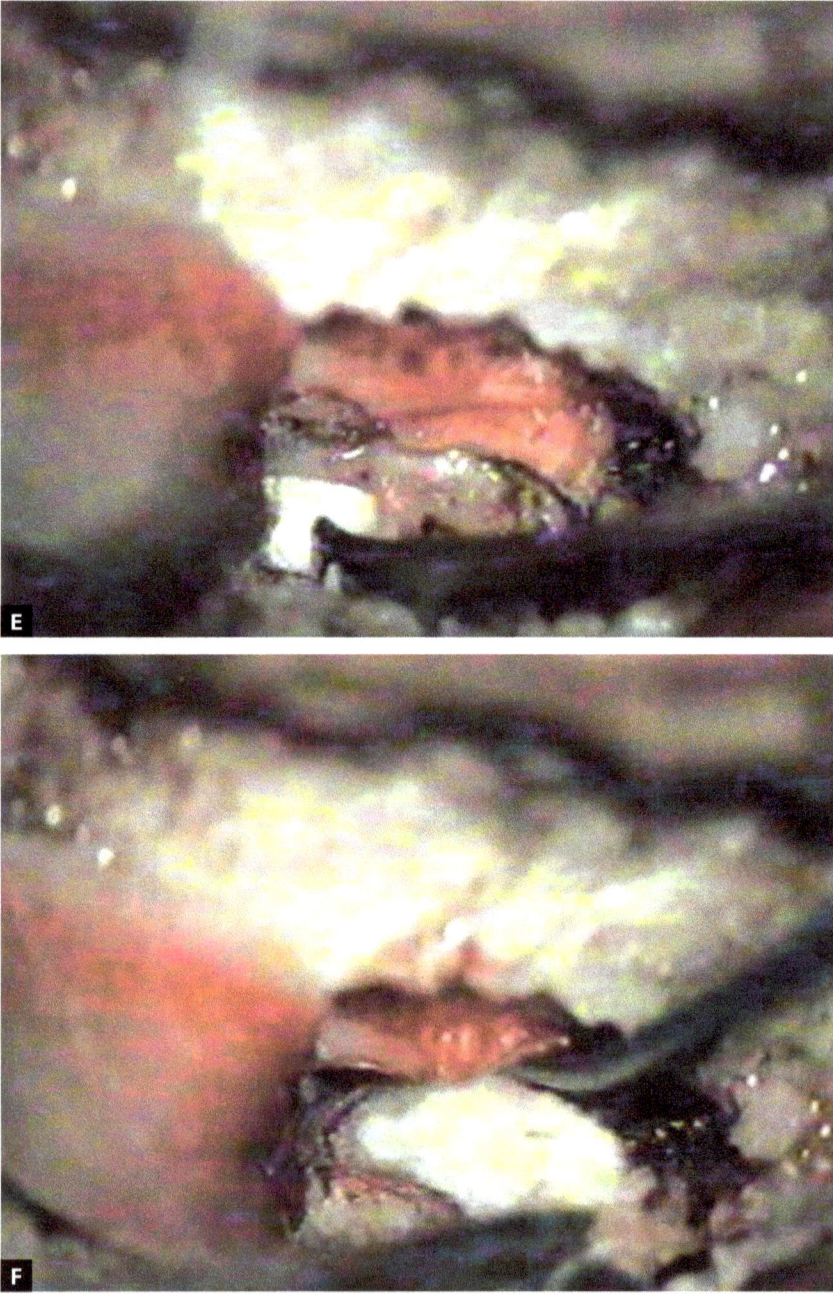

Figs 3.187E and F

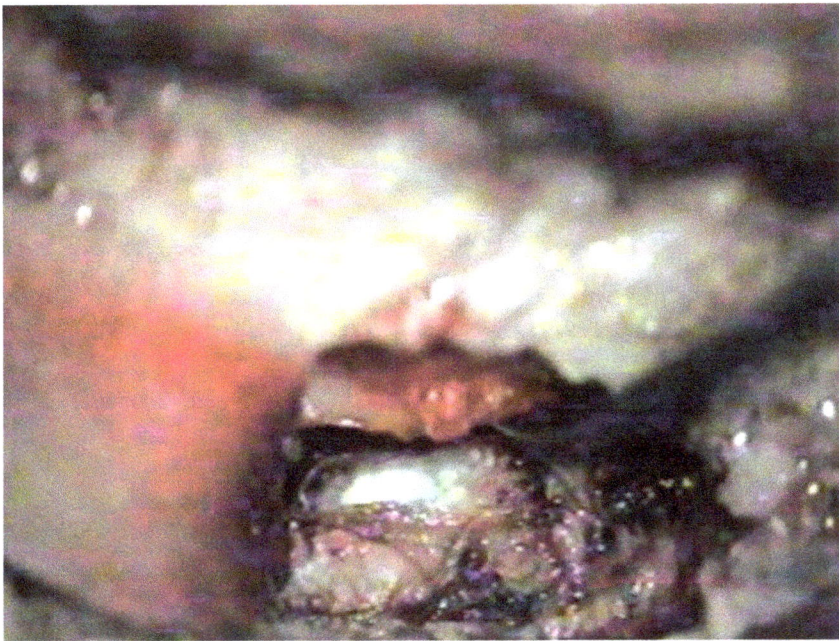

Fig. 3.187G

Figs 3.187A to G: (A) Paraspinal muscle retracted and the lateral edge of the pars exposed; (B) Lateral edge of pars drilled; (C) Trimmed with Kerrison punches; (D) Ligamentum flavum excised, thus foraminotomy performed and the far lateral disc exposed; (E) After opening the annulus, degenerated disc material excised; (F) Nerve root retraction may be necessary during disc material removal; (G) After removal of disc material, intradiscal and epidural search for left small pieces need to be completed

Far-lateral Disc Prolapse (Axillary Approach)

Case Example 2 (Figs 3.188 and 3.189)

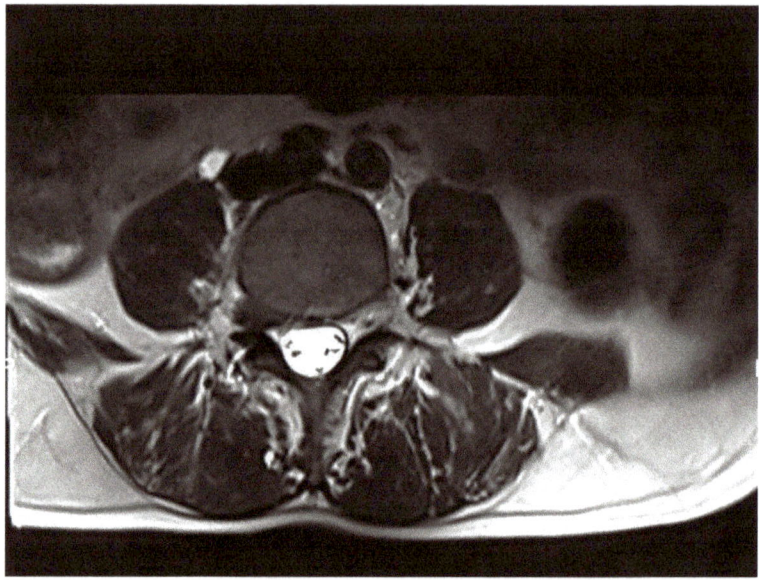

Fig. 3.188 MRI axial cut showing a disc prolapse at foraminal level on right side

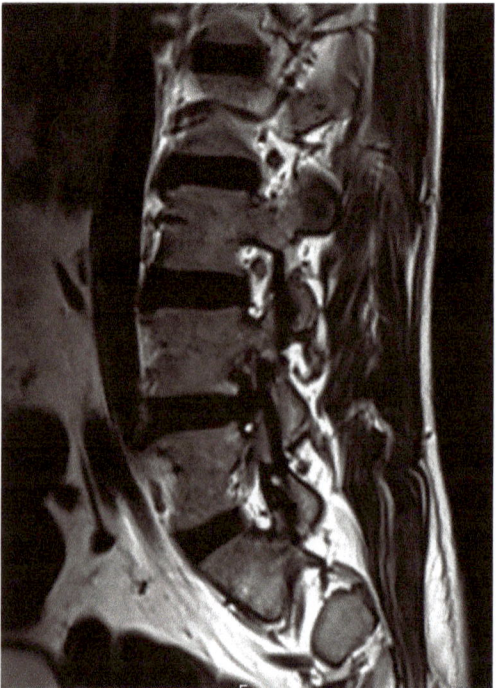

Fig. 3.189 MRI sagittal view showing superiorly migrated disc fragments from L_4/L_5 disc and compressing the nerve root at foramen

Clinical status: Middle aged man complaints of severe pain from his right hip to the knee joint on anterior thigh and lateral aspect of thigh.

Foraminotomy and Discectomy (Axillary Approach)

Operative Procedure

Step 1-Foraminotomy: The paraspinal muscle is dissected and retracted against the spinous process by a double hook retractor exposing pars interarticularis of L_4 vertebra on right side. The inferior facet is well delineated **(Fig. 3.190)**. Lateral border of pars and its inferior edge that continues as the lateral border of inferior facet is drilled out **(Fig. 3.191A)** and subsequently removed with Kerrison punch to complete the bony excision **(Fig. 3.191B)**. Ligamentum flavum is exposed well and the same is removed **(Fig. 3.191C)**.

Step 2-Discectomy: Epidural fat is dissected meticulously and the bulging annulus exposed medial to the nerve root **(Fig. 3.192A)**. Annulus is cut and the degenerated disc fragment hooked out **(Fig. 3.192B)** and removed **(Fig. 3.192C)**. The nerve root is lax and the axillary approach to this disc prolapse is well appreciated **(Figs 3.192D and E)**.

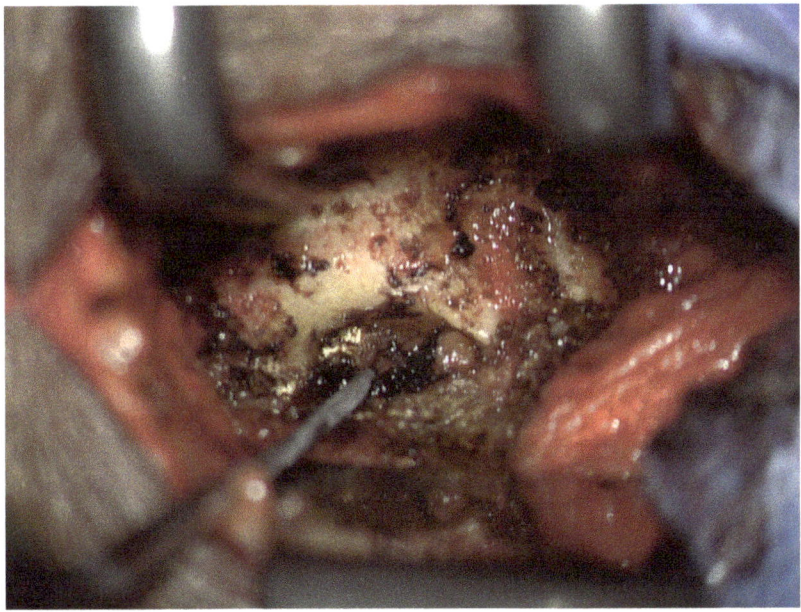

Fig. 3.190 Pars interarticularis exposed

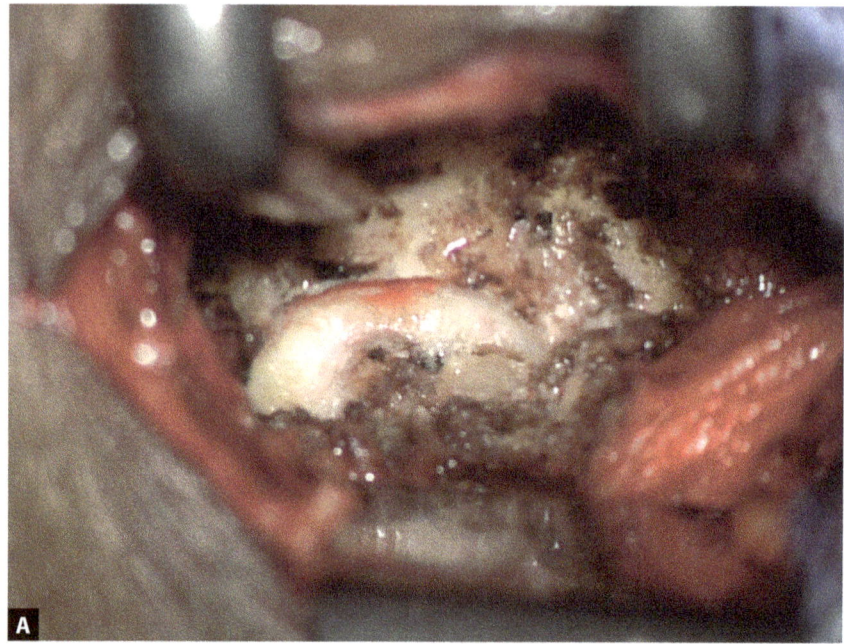
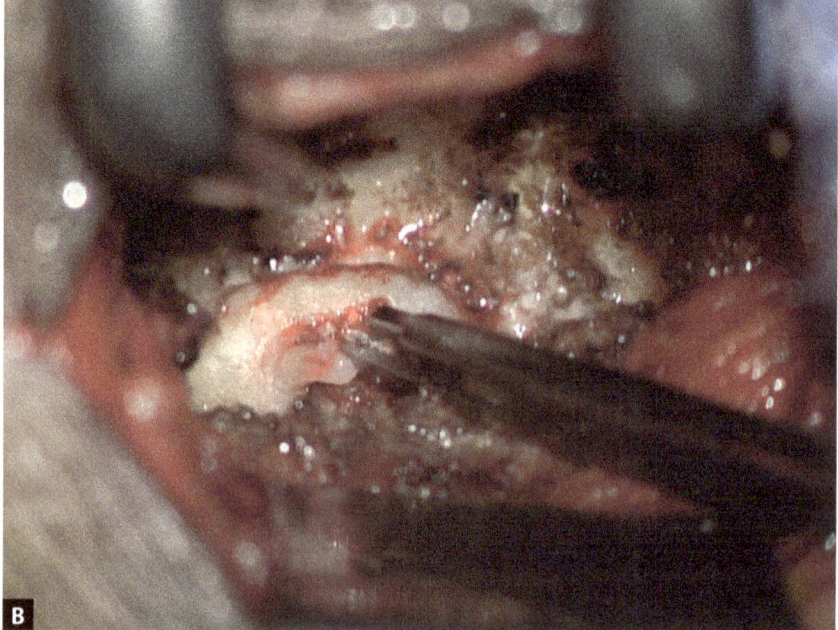

Figs 3.191A and B (A) Lateral edge of pars drilled; (B) Lateral edge of pars excised

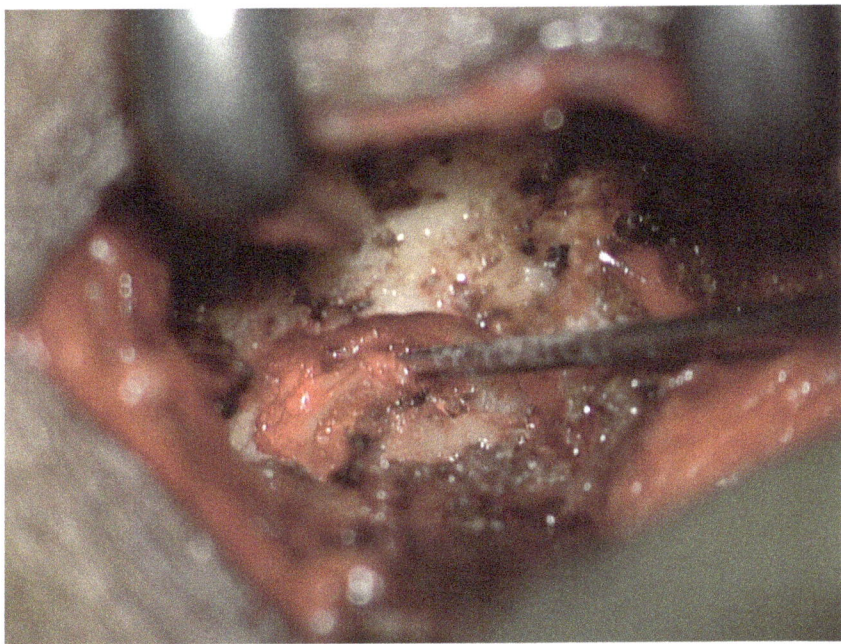

Fig. 3.191C Ligamentum flavum exposed

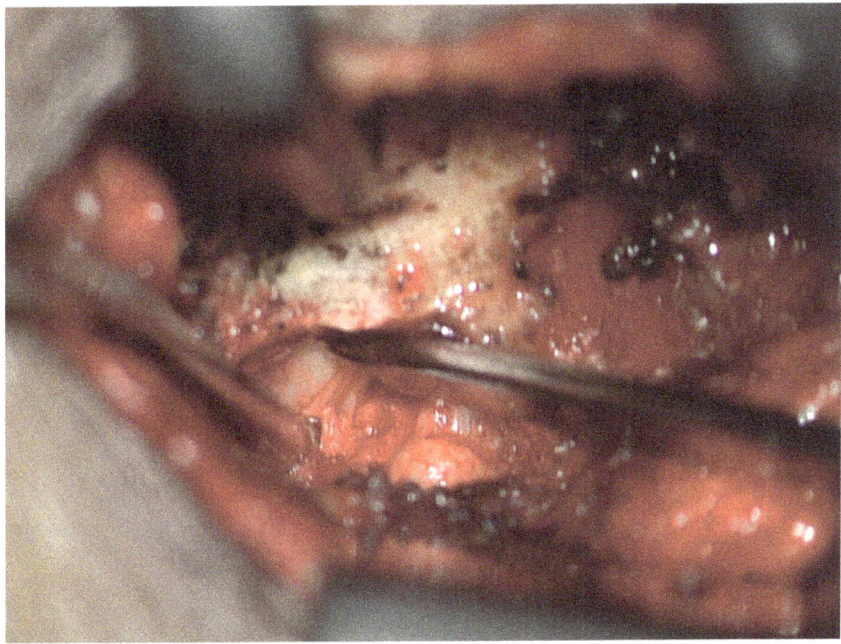

Fig. 3.192A Bulging annulus exposed

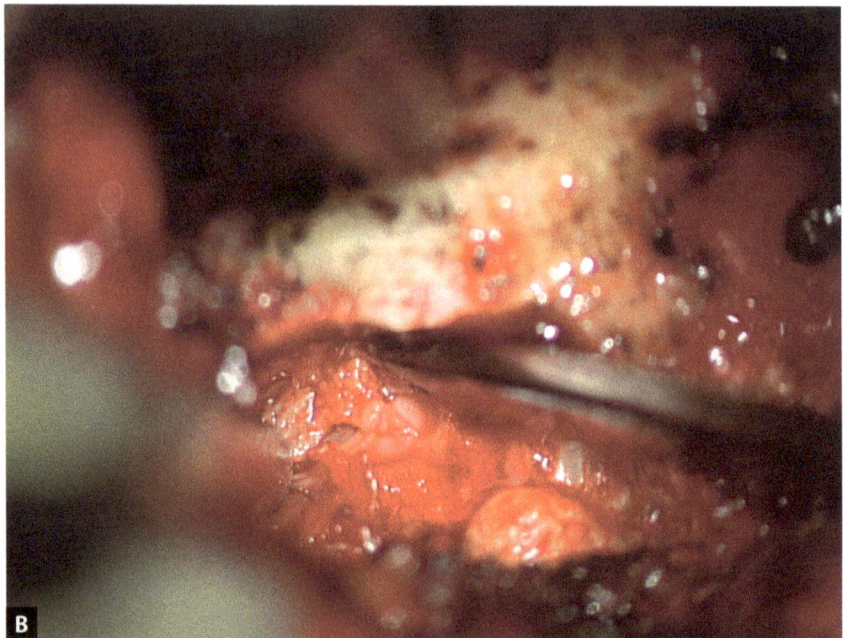

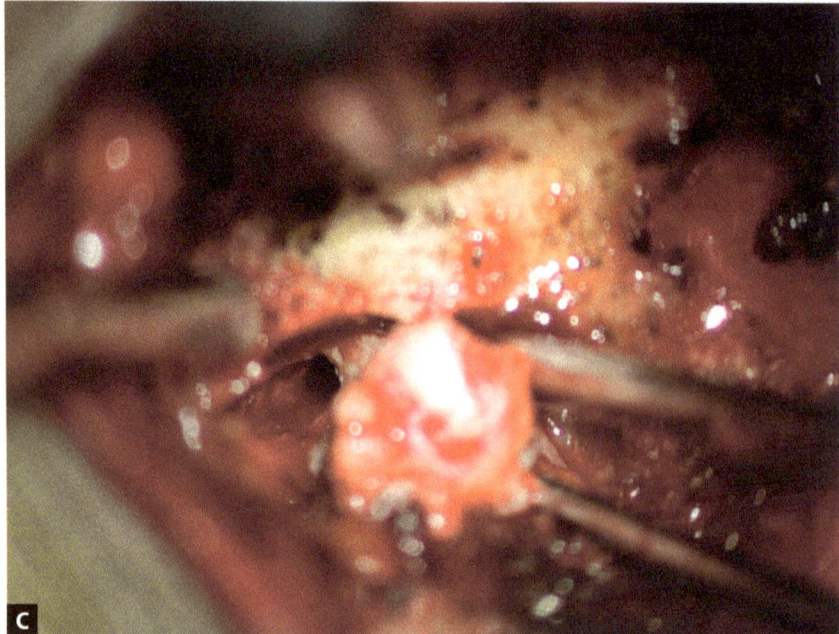

Figs 3.192B and C (B) Annulus opened and degenerated disc material hooked out; (C) Prolapsed disc removed

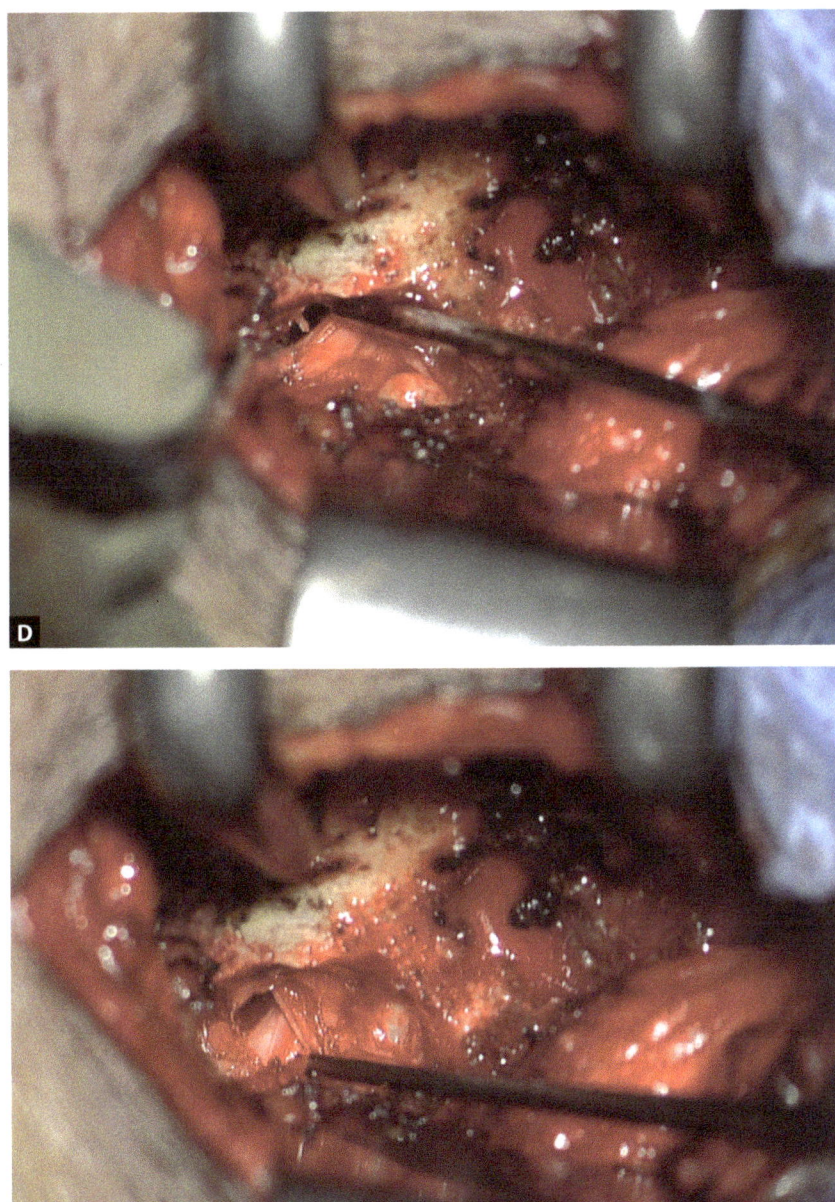

Figs 3.192 D and E (D) Epidural space explored through the axilla of nerve root; (E) Relax nerve root

CHAPTER 4

On-table Complications

On-table complications are very rare in micro lumbar discectomy. As in any other surgery if the principles and basics are strictly followed, they do not occur.

DURAL TEAR

Dural tears are very rare but can lead to cerebrospinal fluid (CSF) leak if unattended. Tears that are visible should be closed using Number 6-0 (0.7 metric) 9 mm, 3/8 circle round bodied or 8-0,8 mm, 3/8 circle taper polypropylene blue monofilament suture material. Meticulous approximation of the dural edge is essential. When the arachnoid is torn, the nerve roots may prolapse through the defect and hence a zero pressure microsuction tube is used to suck the CSF over a small cottonoid on and near the defect to visualize the torn dural edges. The surgical assistance is very important at this stage. Suturing should be preferably done under high magnification **(Figs 4.1 to 4.5)**. Once well-approximated,

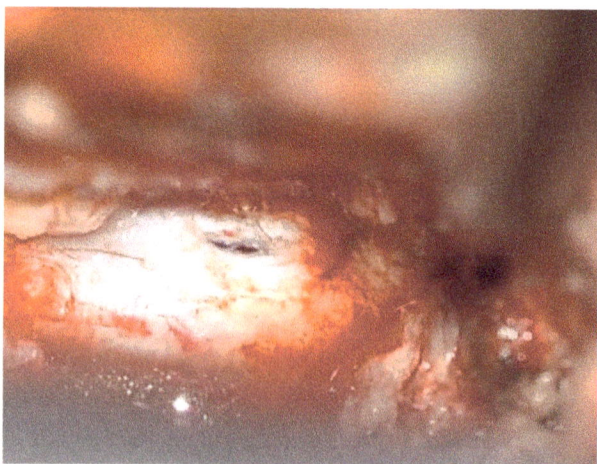

Fig. 4.1 Dural rent seen

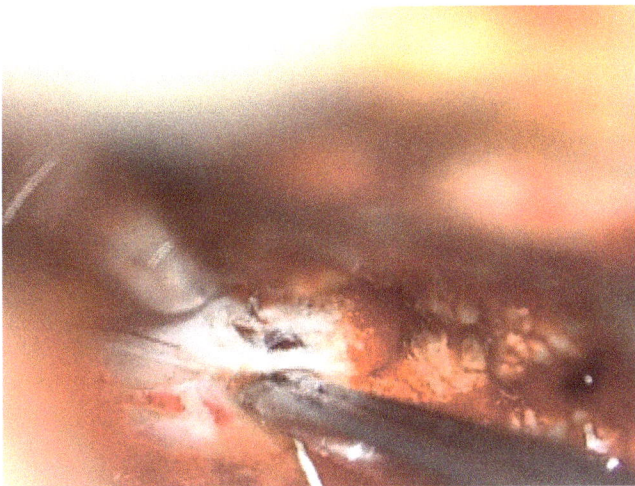

Fig. 4.2 No. 6-0 9 mm suture needle passing through dural rent

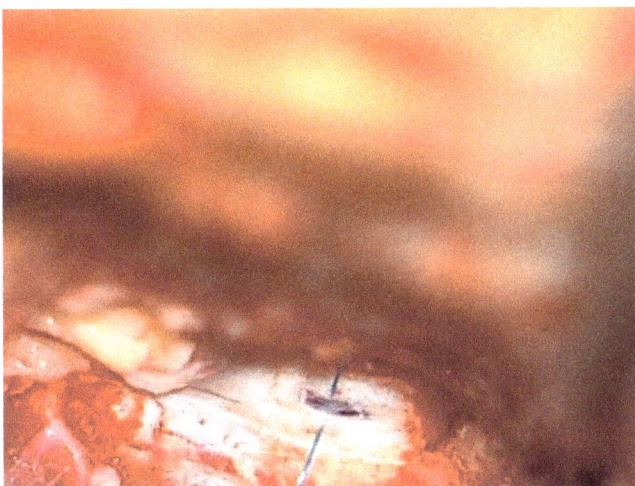

Fig. 4.3 No. 6-0 polypropylene blue monofilament suture material passing through dural rent

CSF leak will stop immediately. In situations where the tear is on the nerve root dural sleeve, then it is very tricky. Defects seen dorsally can be still manageable. However, those that are present laterally or unsuitable for suturing may need patching with fat-lobule harvested from subcutaneous area **(Figs 4.6 and 4.7)**. These fat grafts can be placed over and around the nerve roots and can be fixed with fibrin glue or sealants **(Figs 4.8A to C)**. Mobilizing epidural fat from nearby is always advised. We generously pack over the interlaminar space with fat graft. Muscle patches are not used in

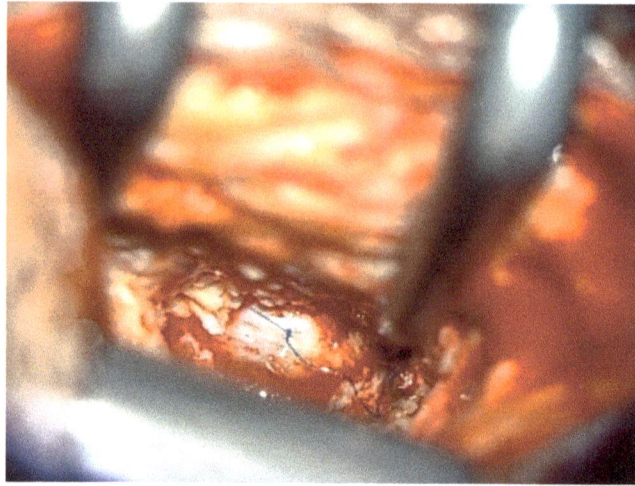

Fig. 4.4 Rent closed and knot secured

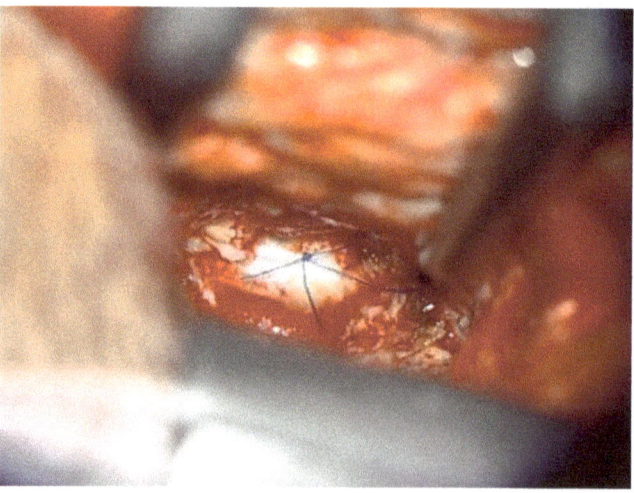

Fig. 4.5 Another suture close to previous suture performed

our practice. Finally the closure is methodical and the fascia closed well. Subcutaneous layer closed with 2-0, 36 mm, 1/2 circle taper polyglactin 910 suture material and subcuticular layer is closed with 3-0,24 mm 3/8 circle, reverse cutting, poliglecaprone suture material. Usually a drain is avoided when the closure is perfect. Mobilizing the patient early in postoperative period avoids CSF leak. Flexion and straining should be avoided in the postoperative period.

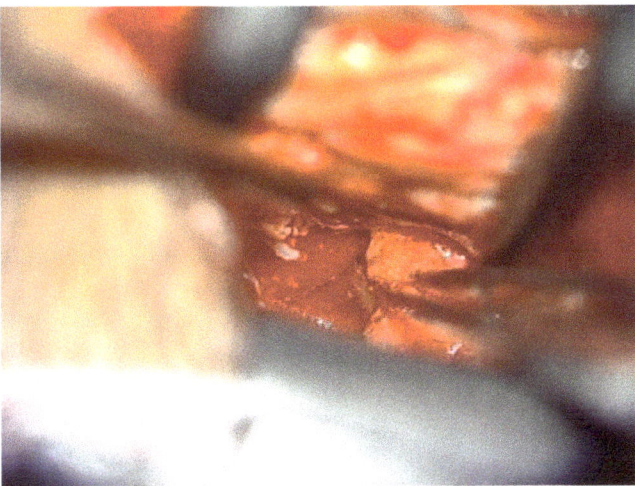

Fig. 4.6 Fat lobules harvested locally from subcutaneous fat tissue

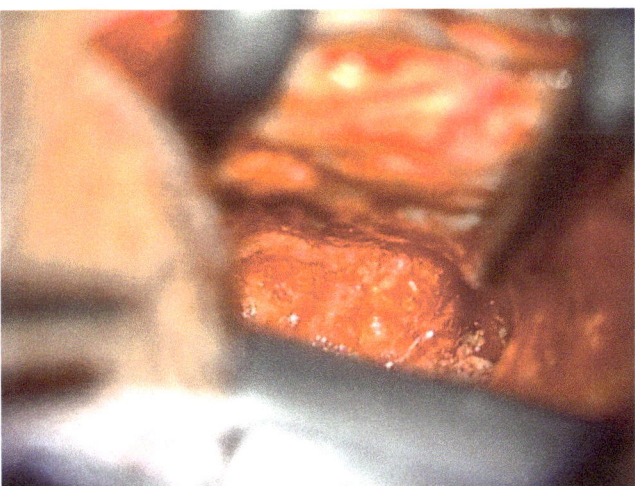

Fig. 4.7 Further fat placed to the entire length

EPIDURAL VENOUS BLEED

Epidural bleeding is frustrating and often disturbs the rhythm of surgery. Usually the veins get breached while retracting the nerve roots medially. It is wise to meticulously cauterize the veins that obstruct visualization of prolapsed disc material and cut them with microscissors to mobilize the plexus away. Low energy bipolar cautery with sharp bipolar tips and micro-bipolar with single probe is used as per the requirement **(Fig 4.9)**.

Surgeon should be patient while achieving hemostasis. If not possible with cautery then hemostats can be used to arrest the bleeder. Gentle pressure over the bleeder with the hemostats held by a small cottonoid and suction tube usually provide good tamponade and finally achieve hemostasis. While doing this, retraction of root and dural sleeve medially should be avoided. Warm saline irrigation also helps in reducing bleeding. Leaving the cottonoids for few minutes usually acheive good hemostasis. Cottonoids and hemostats can then be removed gently and the epidural region be irrigated with warm saline for some time. Never tamponade be done blindly.

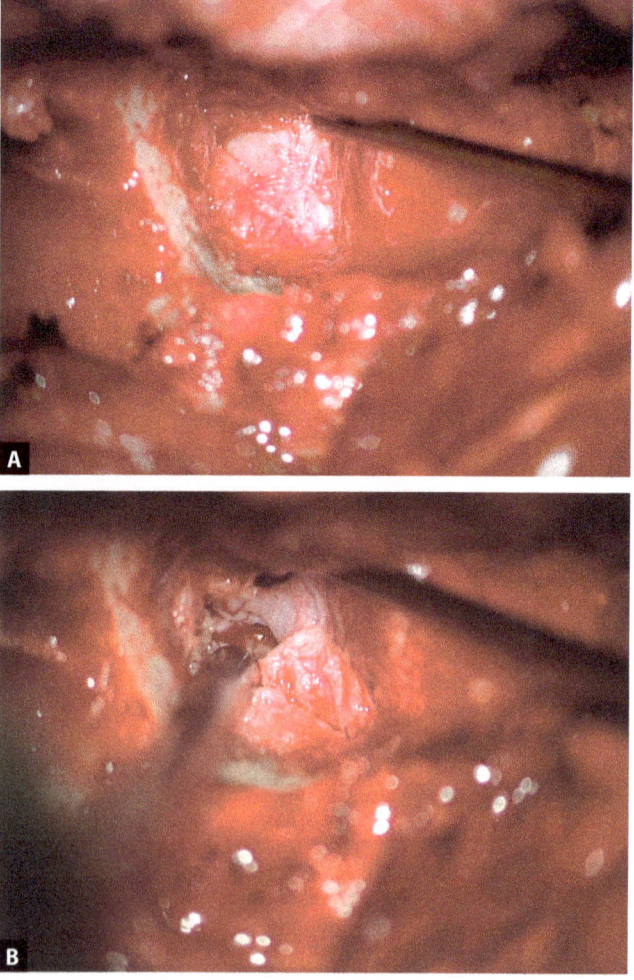

Figs 4.8A and B (A) Perineural fibrosis of nerve root in a case of lateral canal deroofing; (B) Dural rent on the ventral and lateral aspect of nerve root with arachnoid herniation and cerebrospinal fluid leak

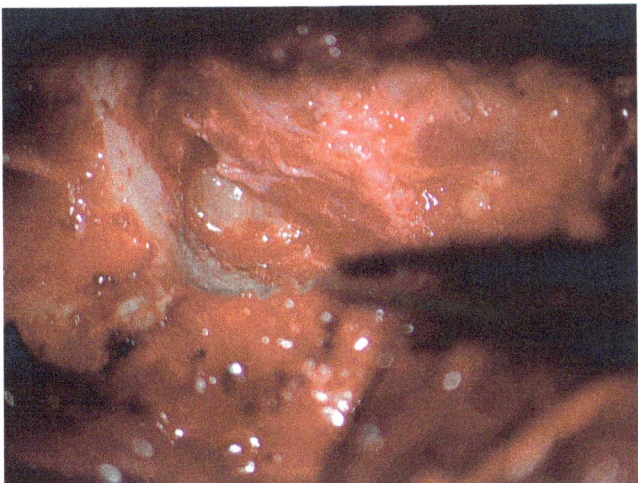

Fig. 4.8C Fat graft placed ventral and lateral over the nerve root. Micro suturing is technically difficult in this condition

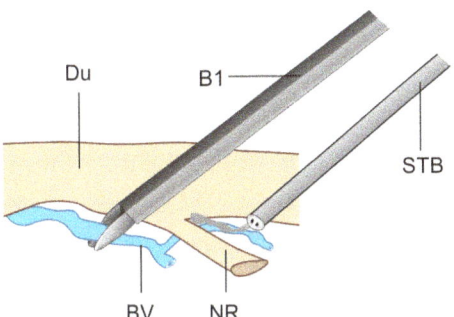

Fig. 4.9 On-table complications
Abbreviations: BV, Batson's venous plexus; B1, Bipolar tips; STB, single tip bipolar; Du, dura; NR, nerve root

A good visualization of nerve root and dura during hemostasis is mandatory and be done under high magnification. Usually, epidural bleeding is observed after removing a large disc material. Surgeons need not get annoyed with this and should deal them with patience. A distended urinary bladder and improperly placed bolsters can increase intra-abdominal pressure resulting in engorged Batson's plexus. This is one important reason I advise the surgeons to ensure a free abdomen while positioning and a temporary urinary catheter during the procedure.

CHAPTER 5

Steps to Prevent Epidural Fibrosis

Once the epidural space is violated, fibrosis tends to follow. However, every attempt should be made to prevent or lessen the chance of postoperative epidural and perineural fibrosis. Less dissection, less cautery, less violation of normal tissue, meticulous handling of nerve root and disc space, good hemostasis, abundant saline irrigation, removal of hemostats at the end, repositioning of nearby epidural fat around the nerve root and dura, installation of epidural steroids, placement of a drain to obtain a dry space after closure, are some of the steps that can prevent fibrosis. Many times we see improperly removed ligamentum flavum adherent with dura. Some times the left out hemostats seen struck to nerve dural sheath. Discitis significantly increases the chance of granulation and inflammatory tissues around the dural sleeves causing fibrosis and intradural adhesions with arachnoiditis. They are difficult to treat and hence need to be prevented.

CHAPTER 6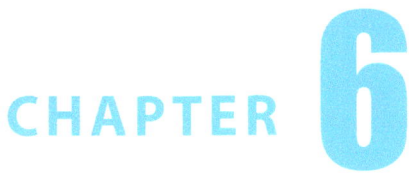

Epidural Medications

Epidural medications are claimed to prevent immediate postoperative pain. Perineural fibrosis, aggravation of existing inflammation and infection. I am not a proponent of this since, in my view, if the surgical technique is gentle and performed well, they are not mandatory. However I have noticed comfortable postoperative period in majority of the patients, where they were used. I am not sure if they really reduce postoperative fibrosis and infection though, they are routinely used in many centers. I advise their use when nerve roots were seen inflamed and in situations where nerve root retraction was considered more than what was required.

One mL of triamcinolone (40 mg steroid) is mixed with one or two mL of bupivacaine 0.25% (long-acting local anesthetic agent) is mixed and instilled over the nerve root and dura after completion of the procedure and allowed to stay over while closure. While bupivacaine 0.25% acts as sensory block, the same agent at 0.50% acts as motor block. Hence, care must be taken to select the correct percentage. Bupivacaine 0.25% is also injected subcutaneously at the incision site for postoperative pain relief.

Saline mixed with antibiotics is used to wash the operative site during the procedure. Vancomycin powder mixed in saline is commonly used. Vintage garamycin is also used.

CHAPTER 7

Micro Lumbar Double-hook Retractors

Ever since the concept of minimal invasiveness came into practice, various types of retractor systems were designed to minimize the tissue damage. Even today, many surgeons use simple right angled Langenberg retractor blades to retract the paraspinal muscles. They are held by an assistant or a nurse and the retraction is intermittent as and when required. Some surgeons use retractors that are held by weight to retract paraspinal muscle.

Single hook retractors are popular. The hook is placed against interspinous ligament and flat blade rest on paraspinal muscle. For a satisfactory exposure the paraspinal muscle needs to be retracted well beyond the facets **(Fig. 7.1)**. This obviously exerts pressure on interspinous ligament and occasionally damages it. Postoperatively, one can appreciate the impression or damage created by the hook on interspinous ligament **(Fig. 7.2)**. This is due to the fact that one needs to retract the paraspinal muscles against an elastic structure that is the interspinous ligament which obviously bear the brunt of retraction force. In my view, ligaments are sensitive to pain and obviously the injured ones produce severe back pain in the immediate postoperative period. Hence it's is better to retract the muscle against bone (lateral surface of spinous process) as done in Homan's retractors. Often single hook on the bone provides oblique exposure. To obviate these limitations, we designed the double-hook system **(Fig. 7.3)**. Instead of single hook on the medial side two hooks are provided so that they can rest on adjacent spinous processes **(Fig. 7.4A)** or on the base of single spinous process **(Fig. 7.4B)** and retract the muscle more efficiently providing wider and stable exposure **(Figs 7.5A and B)**. Injury to interspinous ligament is thus avoided.

There are many claims that separation of paraspinal muscle from bone is the cause for back pain in micro lumber discectomy (MLD). Hence, muscle splitting techniques got introduced. The paraspinal muscles are split by serial dilators and tubular retractors are used to hold them apart during the procedure. It is claimed that when the multifidus fibers are preserved and the muscles are split post-operative backache is less. However, ever since we started using double hook retractors, there was significant reduction in immediate postoperative pain. In general, postoperative back pains are insignificant in micro lumbar discectomy.

Micro Lumbar Double-hook Retractors

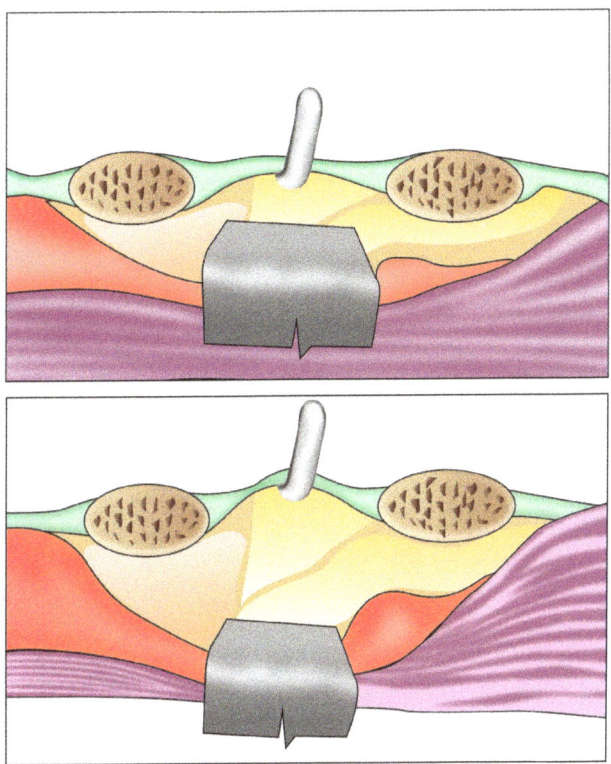

Fig. 7.1 Single-hook system in MLD

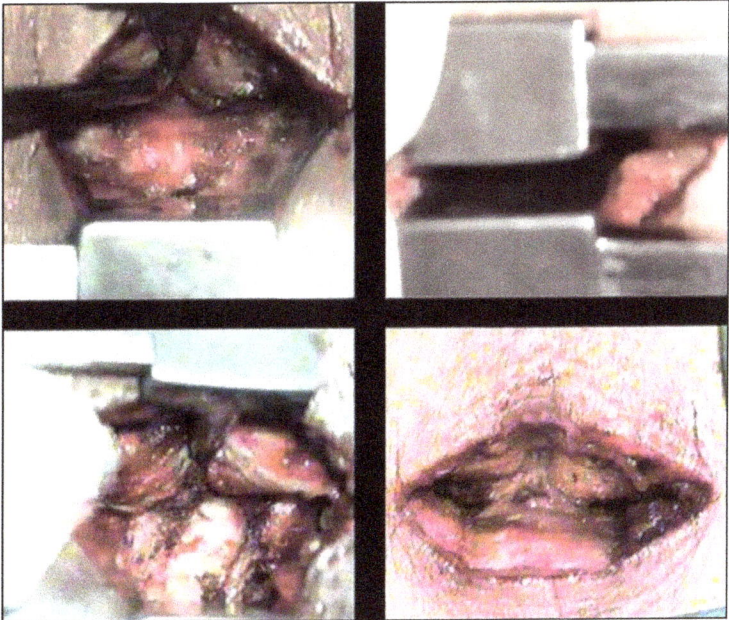

Fig. 7.2 Single-hook stretching interspinous ligament

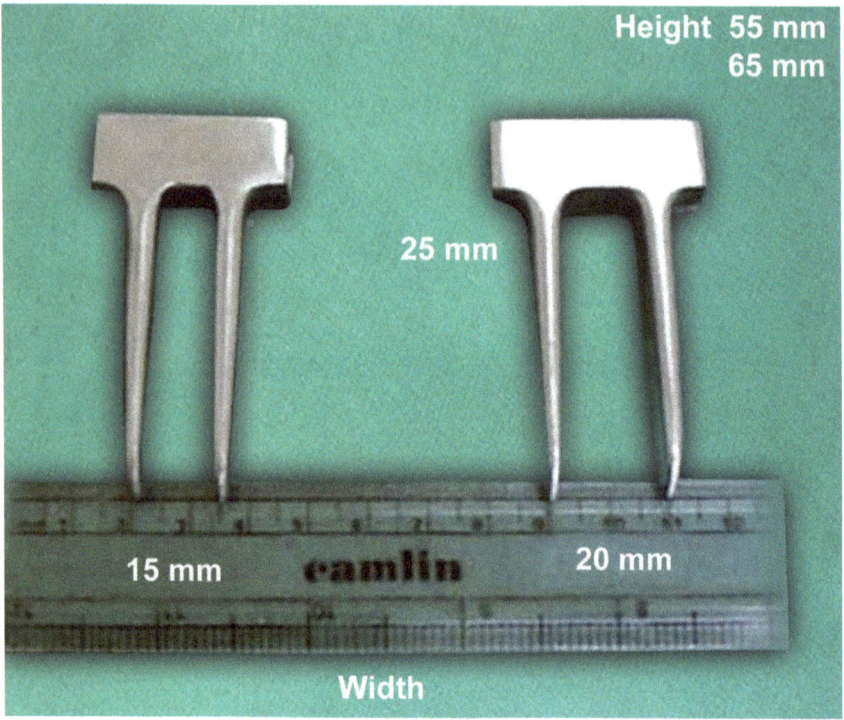

Fig. 7.3 Dr Parthiban double hook

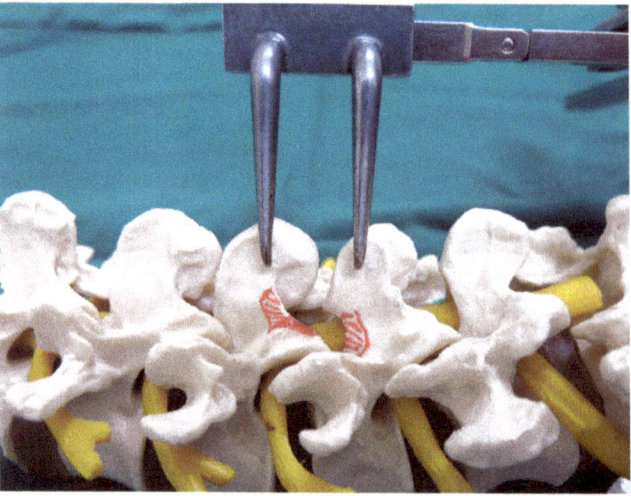

Fig. 7.4A Double hooks rest against adjacent spinous processes

Micro Lumbar Double-hook Retractors | 147

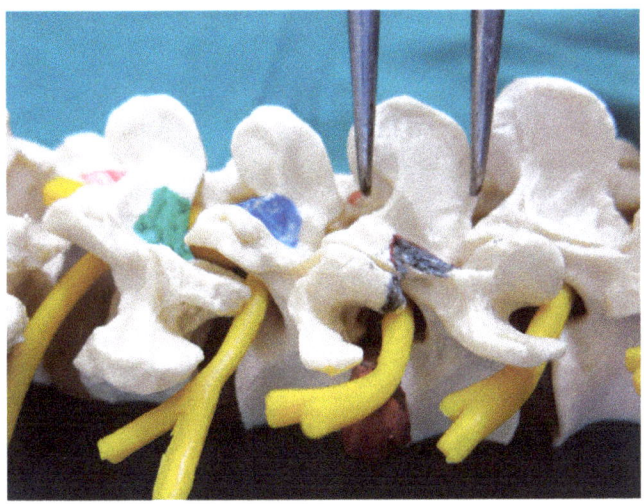

Fig. 7.4B Double-hook rest against single spinous process

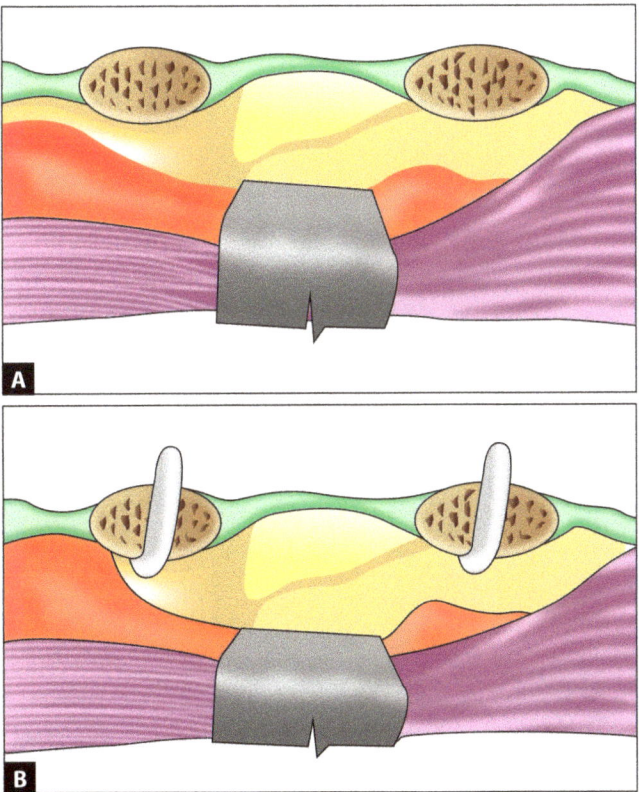

Figs 7.5A and B Double-hook concept: Paraspinal muscles retracted against bone not against ligament

CHAPTER 8

Instruments

Instruments required for micro lumbar discectomy (MLD) are **(Figs 8.1 to 8.13)**:

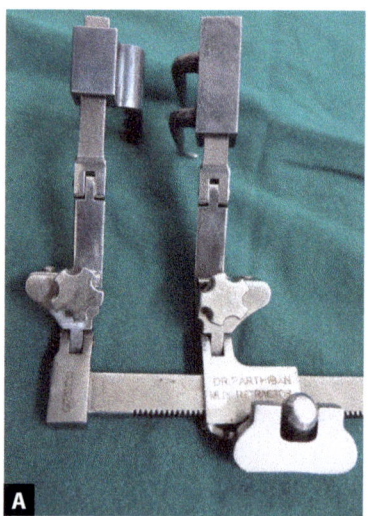

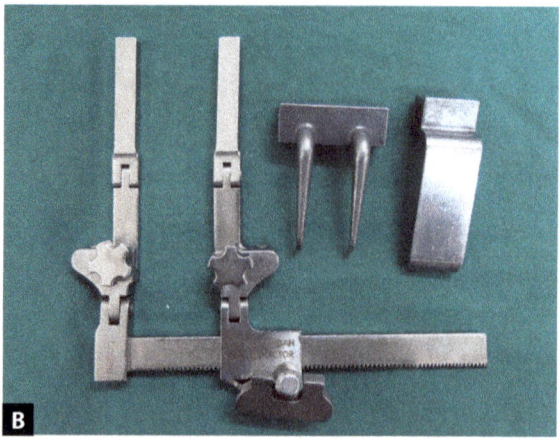

Figs 8.1A and B Micro Lumbar retractor

Instruments | 149

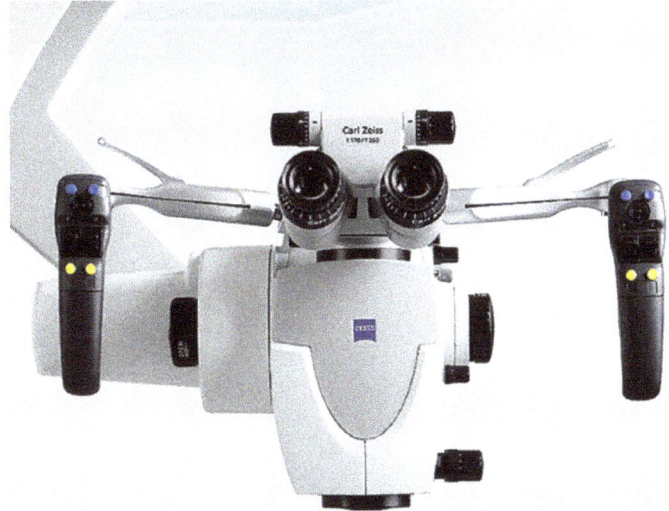

Fig. 8.2 Microscopes

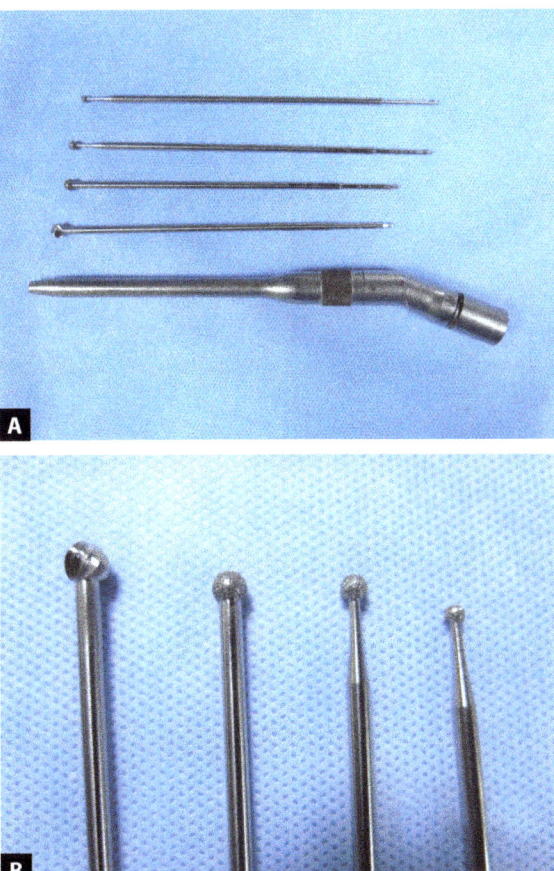

Figs 8.3A and B Micro-angled high-speed drill system

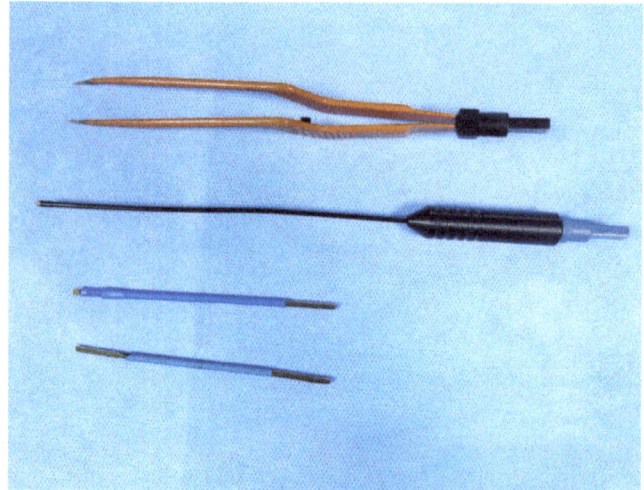

Fig. 8.4 Micro-bipolar and monopolar cautery system

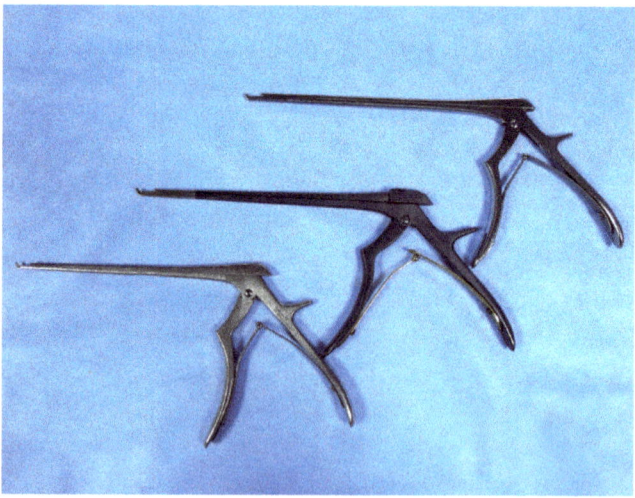

Fig. 8.5 Kerrison punches 45 degree—1 mm, 2 mm, 3 mm, 4 mm

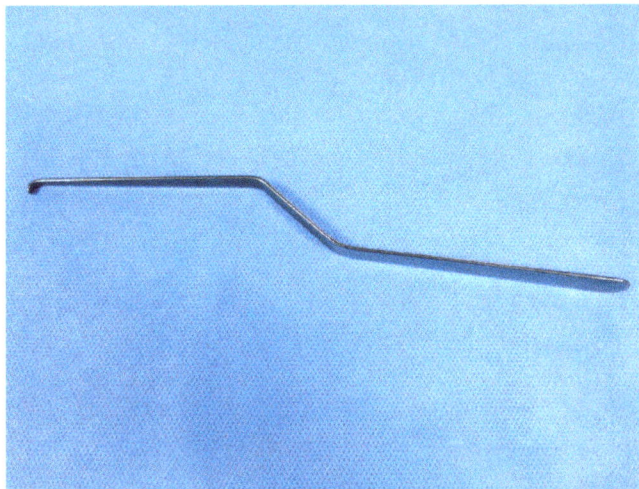

Fig. 8.6 Nerve root retractor

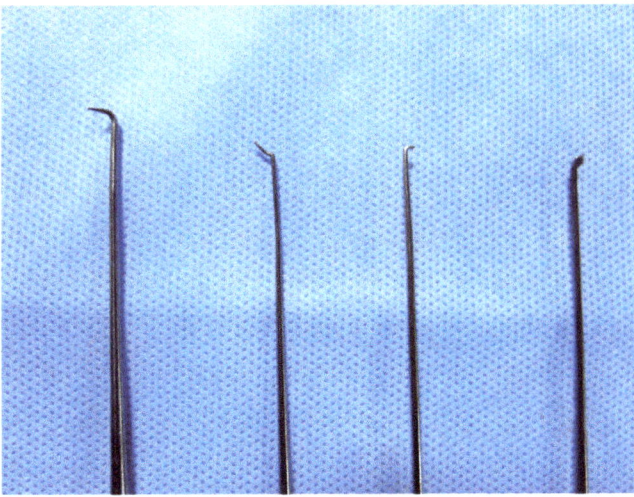

Fig. 8.7 Dissector, Hooks

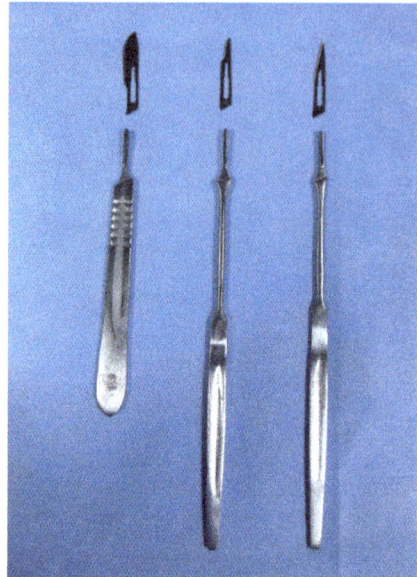

Fig. 8.8 Long handle with Number 11 and 15 blades

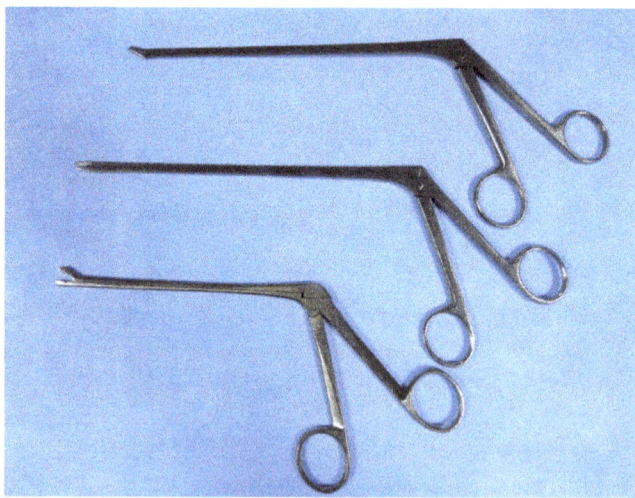

Fig. 8.9 Disc punches

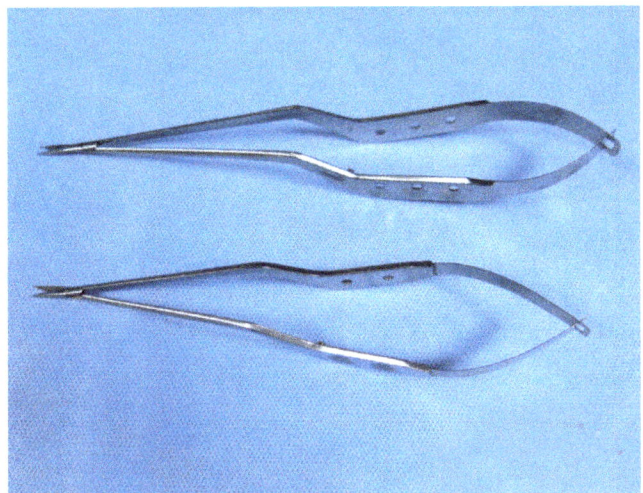

Fig. 8.10 Microscissors

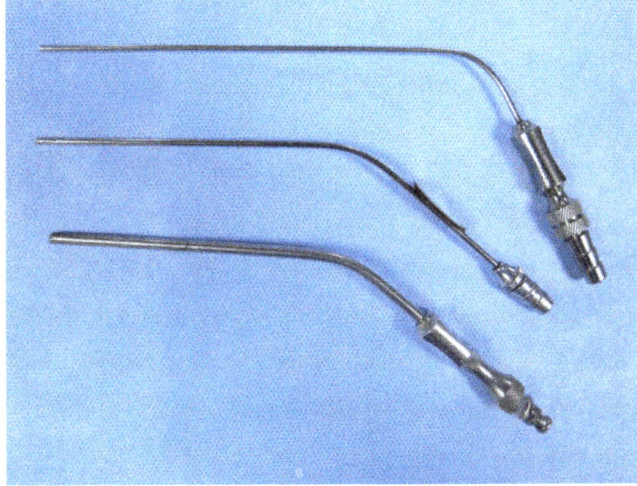

Fig. 8.11 Suction tubes–long

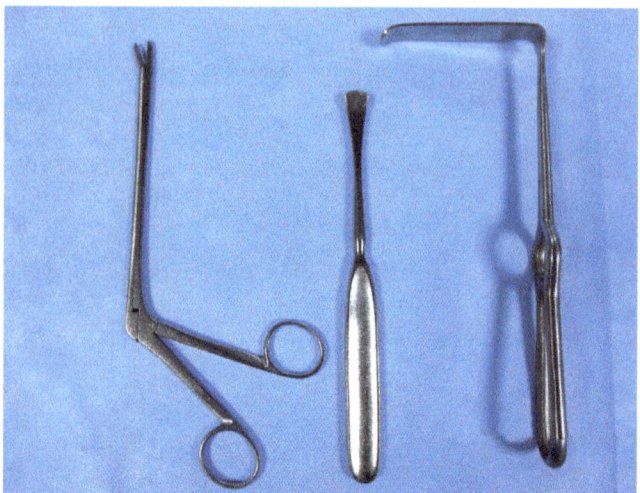

Fig. 8.12 Periosteal elevators, Langenberg retractors, tissue punch

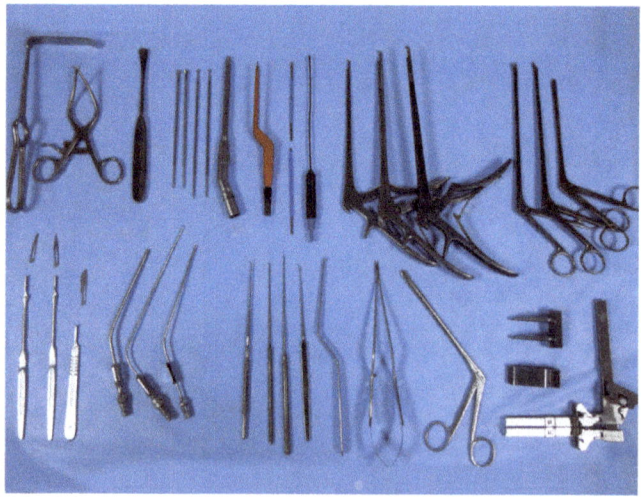

Fig. 8.13 All instruments in a tray

CHAPTER 9

Microscopes and Magnifying Loupes

Microscopes provide stable bright light illumination of operating site with varied magnification. This makes the surgical procedure easy and limits complications due to best visibility the surgeon experiences. Once trained in microsurgery, surgeons do not prefer any other method. However, magnifying loupes with prism lenses of 4× magnification and xenon lights, may be beneficial when microscopes are not available. Loupes need comfort head band and often are very discomfortable. Though I have used them occasionally in the absence of microscopes, I do not recommend them for long period. Microsurgical training is essential **(Figs 9.1 and 9.2)**.

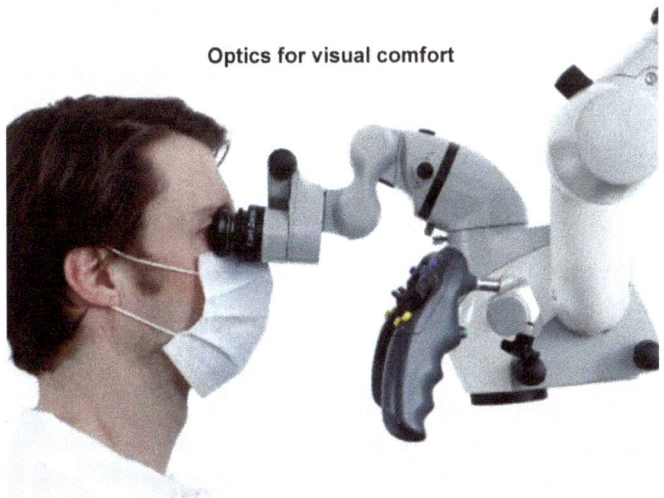

Fig. 9.1 Operating microscope

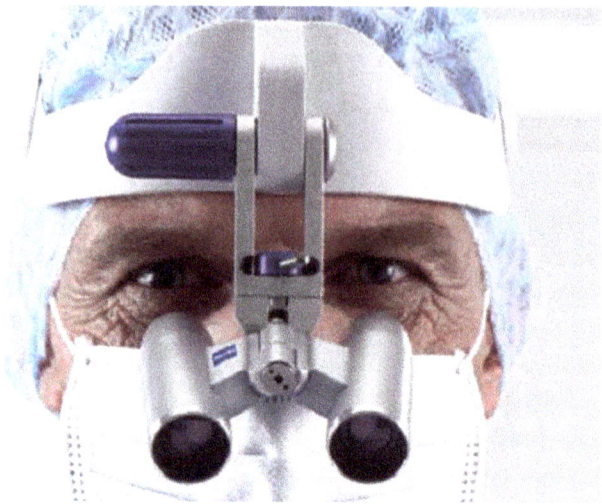

Fig. 9.2 Magnifying loupe

CHAPTER 10

Final Thoughts

Micro lumbar discectomy (MLD) is still considered the gold standard technique and it may take many years to replace it. Ever since it was carved out of laminectomy this technique has claimed good results and has been mastered by many surgeons who were well adept at microsurgery. It is easy to learn and learning curve is acceptably smooth.

In recent times microdiscectomy and those techniques involving para spinal muscle splitting techniques viz. micro endoscopic discectomy and micro discectomy using tubular retractors are grouped under minimal access spinal surgery. The muscle splitting techniques claim advantage over

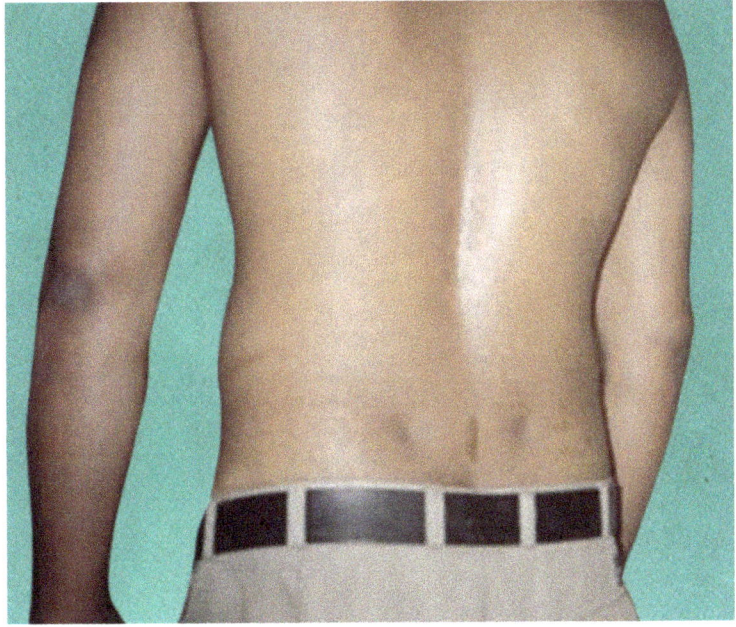

Fig. 10.1 Midline lumbar incision 25 mm is cosmetic

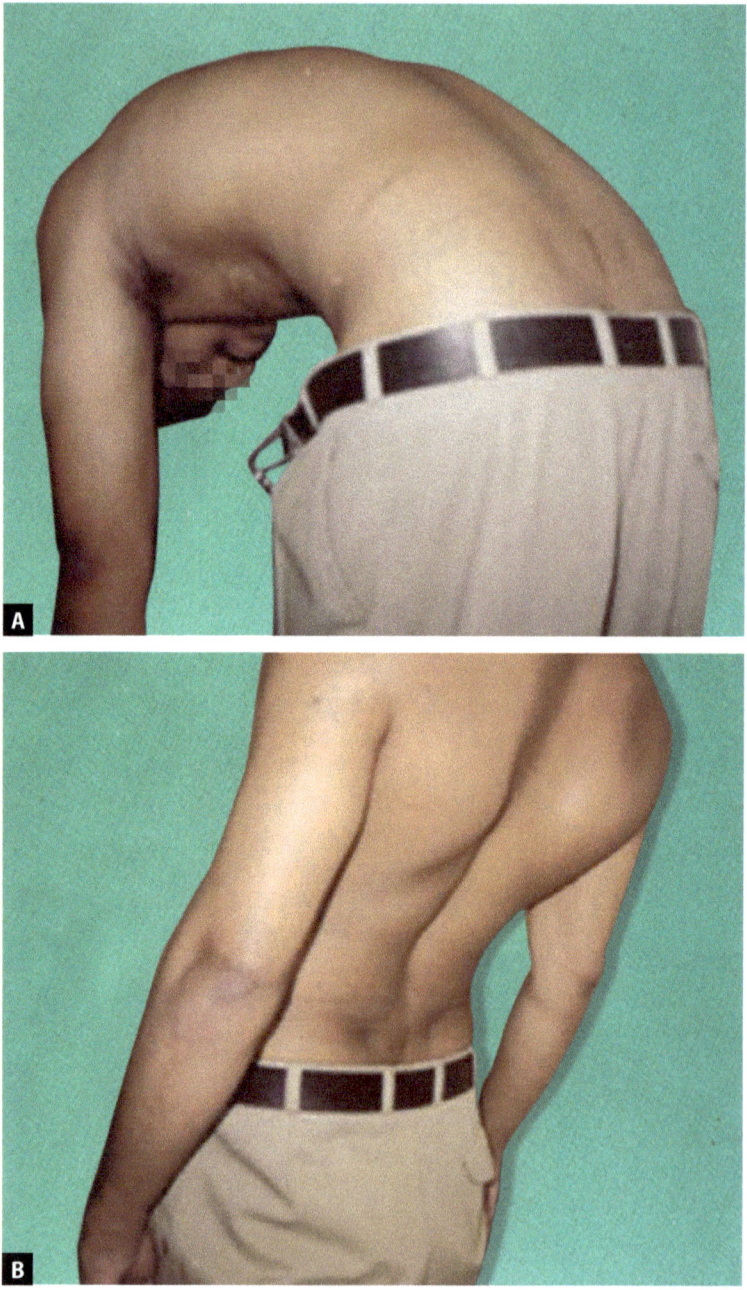

Figs 10.2A and B

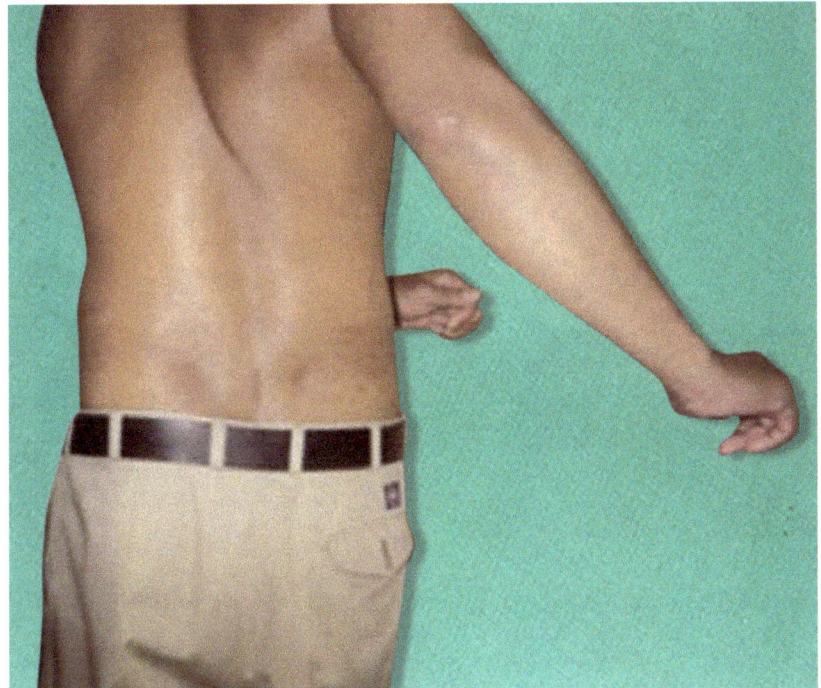

Fig. 10.2C

Figs 10.2A to C (A) Lumbar flexion; (B) Extension: The range of movement offered by micro lumbar discectomy is excellent; (C) Rotation

classical MLD by the so called preservation of paraspinal muscles especially multifidus. The aggressive dissection over laminae by tubular retractor users and inter laminar exposure always make me to think the other way. Single level dissection of paraspinal muscle (unilateral) may not affect the function of multifidus muscle considering its wide and multilevel origin and insertion. Hence, the claim on these retractors in MLD is questionable and do not stand argument. The double hook retractors do not injure the interspinous ligament which is a real concern when a single hook is used to retract the paraspinal muscle against the ligament thus causing strain and pain. Our evidence base is our patients and we enjoy good postoperative function of lumbar spine in our patients **(Figs 10.1 and 10.2A to C)**.

Percutaneous endoscopic discectomy is the only technique (minimally invasive spinal surgery) that does not jeopardise the muscles and ligaments. However, its validity in all varieties of disc prolapses need to be studied. The learning curve is very steep and the technique is still not widely performed at least in this part of the world. Specialists in percutaneous techniques claim

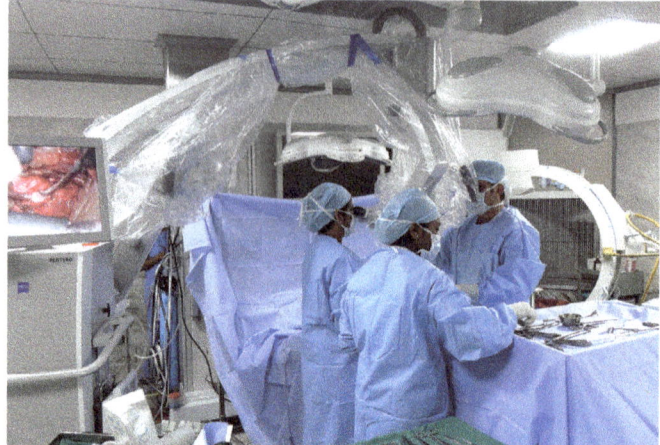

Fig. 10.3 Micro lumbar discectomy is the gold standard

good results and it is obvious that they judiciously use for select cases. It may not match the generosity of utility of micro surgical technique enjoys in lumbar discectomy. We are yet to see the veracity of percutaneous techniques to invade spinal surgery arena. We may hear and see few groups and centers performing them effectively but in general to claim itself as gold standard and to replace the established technique like MLD is a daunting task. Similar views were expressed about MLD many years ago in mid-eighties, comparing that with standard laminectomy. MLD took time to establish due to lack of training in microsurgery among young surgeons. Till then micro lumbar discectomy will stay as gold standard for many more years to come (**Fig. 10.3**). Ultimately, relief of pain and return of function matters for the patient more than the technique alone. That is the reality!

Index

Page numbers followed by *f* refer to figure

A

Annulotomy site 45
Annulus 1, 2, 45
   denervation of 45

B

Batson's venous plexus 4*f*, 5*f*, 55, 141
Bipolar tips 141
Blunt hook 40*f*
Blunt scissors 20*f*
Bolster, diameter of 11*f*
Bony structures, exposure of 99
Bulging annulus 37*f*, 42*f*, 79*f*, 133*f*

C

Canal stenosis, severe 85*f*
Cartilage 1
Cauda equina compression 75*f*
Cavity, abdominal 45
Central disc prolapse 8
Centrolateral large disc prolapse 52

D

Degenerated disc
   fragments 45
   material, superior migration of 98*f*
Disc 5, 45
   bulge 2*f*
   prolapse 8*f*, 17, 53, 76, 86, 93
   punch 45, 152*f*
   space
      exposure of 36
      level of 7*f*
Discectomy 36, 68, 77, 95*f*, 102, 110, 123, 125*f*, 131, 131*f*
   axillary approach 85
   shoulder approach 88
Dorsolumbar fascia 21*f*, 50*f*
Double-hook retractor 50*f*
Dural compression 76*f*
Dural pulsation 83*f*
Dural tear 136

E

Endotracheal intubation 10

Epidual region, exposure of 23*f*
Epidural fibrosis 142
   excision of 120*f*
Epidural space 3
   exposure of 99*f*

F

Facet
   inferior 1, 5, 86, 100, 124
   joint 101*f*
   superior 1, 5, 124
Facetectomy, medial 53, 87*f*, 117*f*
Far-lateral disc prolapse 123, 123*f*, 130
Fascia 22*f*
Fat
   lobules 34*f*
   tissue, subcutaneous 139*f*
Fibrous tissues 121*f*
Flat blade retracts paraspinal muscle 26*f*
Foramen, exposure of 124
Foraminal disc prolapse 8
Foraminotomy 123, 124, 124*f*, 131

G

Ganglion 8

H

Hemostasis 45
Homan's retractors 144

I

Incision 17
Interlaminar space 2, 3*f*, 24*f*
   assessment of 2
   exposure of 17, 53, 76, 86, 107
   widening of 55
Internal vertebral vein 5
Interspinous ligament 4
Intradiscal decompression 42*f*

K

Kerrison punch 31*f*, 64*f*, 94*f*, 102*f*, 117*f*, 129*f*, 150*f*

L

Lamina 2, 17, 53, 76
   inferior 93
   superior 100
Laminectomy edge 100
Langenberg retractors 154
Large disc prolapse 84f, 85f
Lateral canal
   decompression 60f, 77
   stenosis 52
Lateral disc prolapse 8, 16, 17f, 75, 114f
Ligament, lateral part of 32f, 33f
Ligamentum flavum 3, 4, 4f, 25f, 30f, 60f, 62f, 64f, 72f, 87f, 95, 95f, 129f, 133f
Lower lamina, upper border of 29f, 30f
Lumbar
   canal venous drainage 5f
   disc 1, 1f, 2f
   flexion 159f
   neural foramen 5

M

Magnifying loupes 155, 156f
Micro lumbar
   discectomy 144, 148, 157, 159f, 160
   double-hook retractor 26f, 144
Micro-angled high-speed drill system 149f
Microscissors 153f
Microscopes 149f, 155
Micro-tip bipolar cautery 34f
Midline lumbar incision 157f
Migration 84, 98

N

Nerve root 1, 5, 8, 9, 9f, 17, 32f, 47f, 53, 73f, 81f, 87, 87f, 88f, 109f, 111f, 118f, 121f, 135f, 141
   axilla of 135
   axillary region of 96
   compression 17f
   decompression 36, 55, 110
   lateral border of 32f
   perineural fibrosis of 140f
   retractor 9, 17, 47f, 53, 67f, 76, 124, 151f
Neural decompression 102
Neural foramen 1
Nucleus pulposus 1, 2, 8

P

Paraspinal muscle 24f, 129f, 147f
Paraspinal retraction 125f
Pars interarticularis 131
Pedicle 1, 5, 8
Percutaneous endoscopic discectomy 159
Periosteal elevators 154f
Posterior longitudinal ligament 8, 22, 43f

R

Radicular artery 5
Recurrent disc
   fragments 112f
   prolapse 105, 106f, 107f, 113, 114f, 115f

S

Sacral lamina 94f
   superior border of 86f
Sacrum 3
Sciatica 92, 113
Shoulder
   approach 86, 123
   exposure of 115
Single-tip bipolar 141
Single-hook stretching interspinous ligament 145f
Skin
   incision 18f
   marking 18f
Spinolaminectomy 98f
Spinous process 1, 2, 5, 76
Sub-annular degenerated disc fragment 119f
Sub-annular disc prolapse 8f
Subcutaneous bleeders, bipolar cautery of 19f
Suction tubes 153f
Supraspinous ligament 4

T

Tissue
   forceps 24f
   punch 154f

U

Upper lamina, lower border of 28f
Upper vertebra, inferior facet of 56f

V

Veins, epidural 3, 5
Ventral compression 66f
Vertebral body 1, 4, 5, 8

www.ingramcontent.com/pod-product-compliance
Lightning Source LLC
Chambersburg PA
CBHW040540220526
45473CB00016B/2984